The Good Caregiver

The Good Caregiver

A One-of-a-Kind Compassionate Resource for
Anyone Caring for an Aging Loved One

Robert L. Kane, M.D.

with Jeannine Ouellette

AVERY
a member of
Penguin Group (USA) Inc.
New York

AVERY

Published by the Penguin Group

Penguin Group (USA) Inc., 375 Hudson Street, New York, New York 10014, USA • Penguin Group
(Canada), 90 Eglinton Avenue East, Suite 700, Toronto, Ontario M4P 2Y3, Canada (a division of Pearson
Penguin Canada Inc.) • Penguin Books Ltd, 80 Strand, London WC2R 0RL, England • Penguin Ireland,
25 St Stephen's Green, Dublin 2, Ireland (a division of Penguin Books Ltd) • Penguin Group (Australia),
250 Camberwell Road, Camberwell, Victoria 3124, Australia (a division of Pearson Australia Group Pty Ltd) •
Penguin Books India Pvt Ltd, 11 Community Centre, Panchsheel Park, New Delhi–110 017, India •
Penguin Group (NZ), 67 Apollo Drive, Rosedale, North Shore 0632, New Zealand (a division of Pearson
New Zealand Ltd) • Penguin Books (South Africa) (Pty) Ltd, 24 Sturdee Avenue, Rosebank,
Johannesburg 2196, South Africa

Penguin Books Ltd, Registered Offices: 80 Strand, London WC2R 0RL, England

Most Avery books are available at special quantity discounts for bulk purchase for sales promotions, premiums,
fund-raising, and educational needs. Special books or book excerpts also can be created to fit specific needs.
For details, write Penguin Group (USA) Inc. Special Markets, 375 Hudson Street, New York, NY 10014.

Library of Congress Cataloging-in-Publication Data

Kane, Robert L., date.
The good caregiver : a one-of-a-kind compassionate resource for anyone caring for an
aging loved one / Robert L. Kane with Jeannine Ouellette.
p.   cm.
Includes bibliographical references and index.
ISBN 978-1-58333-422-5
1. Older people—Care.   2. Caregivers.   I. Ouellette, Jeannine.   II. Title.
HV1451.K36   2011   2010036955
649.8084'6—dc22

Printed in the United States of America
3   5   7   9   10   8   6   4   2

Book design by Michelle McMillian

To my sister, Candy,

who taught me what caring was really about

Contents

Introduction

The Good Caregiver

Lessons Learned from a Broken System

Long-term care . . . affects a large portion of the population, it is expensive (it currently accounts for about 10 percent of all health care costs), and it requires a unique partnership between government and citizens. Moreover, a range of constituencies perceive the current long-term care system as seriously broken. It exposes people who need services to considerable financial risk, and it too often relies on an institutional model of care that is at odds with consumer preferences.

—David G. Stevenson, Ph.D.,
The New England Journal of Medicine, May 8, 2008

We don't think about long-term care until it hits us in the face. But avoidance is no defense. The average American who lives to age sixty-five has about a 40 percent chance of spending time in a nursing home. As former first lady Rosalynn Carter once said, "There are only four kinds of people in this world: Those who have been caregivers; those who currently are caregivers; those who will be caregivers; and those who will need caregivers." Nearly all of us will have to deal with long-term care either for ourselves or for parents, relatives, friends, or neighbors. But if long-term care is an inescapable consequence of a longer-lived society, why don't we prepare for it?

Partly, it is because we don't get many chances to practice. Except for jokes about it, old age isn't a common dinner party topic. Elder care, dementia, and death aren't things we normally chat about. Even if we did want to educate ourselves, we aren't sure where to turn for sound information or advice. And most of us don't think that far ahead. We rarely read instruction manuals for new appliances unless we can't get the damn things to work. What we usually want is a good index that will direct us to solutions for problems as they arise. That is what this book is designed to do.

Prepare to Care

From the very start, you will need to assess your own or your family's ability to provide care. Chapter One, Becoming a Caregiver, includes a helpful quiz to get you started in assessing your areas of strength and weakness as a care provider. The quiz can also help you identify if you're just not cut out to handle the demands of being a caregiver. Not everyone has the temperament or resources for long-term caregiving. Caregiving is hard and demanding work, but there are lifelong rewards. You will form special relationships in intensely personal and meaningful ways. You will make the lives of people you love immeasurably better. Many, many caregivers speak powerfully to the multiple ways caring for a loved one enriched their own lives and provided a lasting and indelible sense of purpose and meaning.

A Balanced View

In *The Good Caregiver*, I present a balanced view of caregiving, but I do not pull any punches. You will find truthful accounts and practical advice about a world that most people have never before encountered until they find themselves in the middle of it. But you'll also get a glimpse through the usually covered window of long-term caregiving for the elderly, a world where the demands are intense, yes, but where the bonds of love and the memories of powerful shared experience with a loved one at life's most vulnerable juncture can be profoundly transformative.

GIFTS AND LESSONS OF CAREGIVING

- **The realization that the finite nature of our human lives is a gift.** This realization is a compelling motivator not to put off one's dreams, not to stand for a life that is not being fully lived.
- **The deepening of faith.** Faith not necessarily as religion, but as a deeper spiritual connection to the force of life that is universal and enduring.
- **The reconnection with siblings.** Although sibling relationships are often strained in the face of the stress of dealing with a dying parent and perhaps also with unresolved issues of childhood, siblings may get closer and communicate positively and affirm each other more.
- **The wonder of friends.** My friends' concern and small acts of kindness for my mother and for me constituted a beautiful gift.
- **The (growing) ability to say "no."** I had to say no to many things. Some I was fine with; other things were very difficult.
- **The up close and personal view of why it is important to make plans for aging or declining years.** I now understand how important it is to (1) downsize one's material possessions and home; (2) understand one's own social and support network; (3) adapt one's living space for an aging body; and (4) put aside money to serve as a home-based services fund and/or for purchasing long-term care insurance.
- **The growing awareness to invest more time on one's own physical health.** This means the right food, the right exercise, the right sleep.
- **A greater ability to "not sweat the small stuff."**
- **The appreciation of relationships, especially with the person who is in need.**
- **The awareness of the importance of humor.** This comes often by finding the lighter side of a dark event.

—DEB PAONE, CAREGIVING DAUGHTER

How to Use This Book as an Instruction Manual

Most people facing the caregiving role are neophytes. They have never experienced such a challenge before. Knowing how to respond to the nitty-gritty realities of caring for an older person doesn't usually come automatically. New caregivers need a staggering amount of honest, straightforward advice on the nuts and bolts of managing care for a loved one. They need straight talk about the behind-the-scenes tasks that can make a lasting impact on the quality of the caregiving experience for everyone involved. Most people even need step-by-step instructions on handling some of the hands-on caregiving tasks that an older person will need. How do you assist a frail elderly person with bathing? What is the best (and worst) way to deal with urinary incontinence? Is there a simple, safe way to keep track of multiple prescriptions? No one is born knowing the ins and outs of caregiving! Few want to take a course in it.

Ideally, people coming new to caregiving would stop and read the instruction manual from cover to cover. But in my experience, whenever I get a new device with clear instructions to read the whole manual before attempting to operate it, I never do. In fact, I know very few people who do. What most of us want is a good index where we can turn when we run into a problem. This book was written and organized to be used for just that purpose, to be consulted as a resource and guide in the manner that best suits your needs as they arise.

So if you have just found yourself thrown into the role of caregiver, with practically no warning or preparation, you can use this book like the instruction manual for that appliance that would not turn on; just go straight to the chapter that deals with the issue you're trying to deal with *right now*. For example, the nursing home calls to tell you that Mom has some troubling symptoms and is being sent to the emergency room. Before you jump in the car to meet her there (and you should do just that, if you live nearby and are able to), you should review the section on Emergency Rooms in Chapter Eight: Handling Hospitals. Or, maybe there have been some warning signs that are causing you to worry about the safety of your parent's driving. Chapter Five: Daily Life includes everything you need to know about when and how to break the news to Mom or Dad about the end of driving (and you may be surprised that it is often better if you are not the one to deliver this sensitive message). Whether your question is about guardianship, nutrition, adult day care, or hospice, you can use the index at the back of this book to take you straight to the chapters and pages that will answer your immediate questions.

Meanwhile, every chapter contains charts, checklists, and sidebars to help you find what you need easily and quickly. Just as important, you will find the true stories of many other courageous caregivers who've been where you are, and who've learned valuable lessons from their own challenges and mistakes. You may discover that these first-person accounts of caregiving are your greatest source of solace in navigating an unfamiliar and very demanding new role. From the heartfelt stories of others, you will find not just advice, but hope and encouragement for your ability to be a good caregiver despite your uncertainties. And every chapter wraps up with a list of the most important points to ponder— zeroing in on that chapter's essential new information and advice.

How to Use This Book as an Essential Planner

As soon as you can spare the few hours to do so, you should try to scan through this book cover to cover, in order to get the full scope of what you may encounter and what you need to prepare for when it comes to caring for your elderly loved one during his or her last years. The Boy Scouts are right; it is better to be prepared. Investing the time and energy in looking ahead and making the preparations for quality care, including learning the facts about institutional living, since that may very well become a necessity, is absolutely critical in order to avoid making hasty decisions later, in times of crisis. As you will see in Chapter Ten: Moving Time, the more time you take to think ahead about critical milestones and transitions in caregiving, the less likely you will be to rush into a bad decision in the midst of a crisis.

At every juncture in a caregiving journey, you will find yourself faced with the task of understanding new and complex legal and financial information and options, often with little time to make sound choices. That is why the first three chapters of this book offer detailed advice and resources on the many concrete and complex tasks of managing care for the person you love. After Chapter One's thorough overview on becoming a caregiver, Chapter Two: Money and the Law addresses the basics of what you need to know about the financial and legal aspects of overseeing your loved one's medical care. Chapter Three focuses exclusively on the crucial task of finding the right doctor for your aging parent. With the particular and specific health challenges of aging and the tremendous shortage of geriatricians, finding the right doctor may be harder than you'd have guessed. At the outset of your journey of caregiving, you must also prepare for the necessity of caring for yourself, even when it does not seem practical or even possible to do so. Caregiving is hard work, and can be dangerous when the caregiver's own basic needs are not met. Chapter Four outlines several practical, proven strategies for approaching long-term caregiving as a marathon, not a sprint, and preparing yourself accordingly. By recognizing the risks of ignoring your needs and by following some sound advice, you can avoid a collapse and see to it that you will have the stamina to go the distance.

Chapter Five: Daily Life steers you through all of the basics of daily caregiving, from bathing and dressing to eating and exercise. A good caregiver has to know how to provide the right amount of care without "overcaring," so that the loved one is able to maintain as much autonomy and dignity as possible. Knowing when to worry and when to let go, when to intervene and when to step back, is an art and a science that Chapter Five helps explain in plain English. Likewise, the common ailments of aging and their treatments can present challenges for caregivers. When does a decreased appetite require attention? What are the indications that an ache or pain requires treatment? Chapter Six provides the information you need to help your loved one live as safely as possible, with the most functionality and the least pain.

Often, one of the greatest fears caregivers face is the onset of dementia in an aging parent or a spouse. And rightfully so. Caregivers of persons with dementia certainly experience high rates of stress and even illness related to their caregiving. Alzheimer's disease and other maladies of the aging brain require specialized understanding and a great deal of perspective, patience, humor, and skill. Indeed, dementia and its challenges may be more fear-provoking than any other element of long-term caregiving. All of this is discussed in detail in Chapter Seven.

Chapter Eight provides what you never knew but will need to understand about hospitals in order to be an effective caregiver. While hospitals are places of healing, they pose particular stresses for elderly patients, and the more you know about those stresses, the better able you will be to ask the right questions and steer clear of the most common pitfalls of hospital stays for older persons. You cannot assume that hospital personnel will always do the right things or follow through on your requests. From admission to discharge and every step in between, including the special considerations of emergency room visits for the frail patient, Chapter Eight includes tips about what to watch for and how to advocate for your loved one in the event a hospital stay becomes necessary.

By now, you are already getting a sense of the enormity of a caregiver's job. But you should also be getting the sense that caregiving for an elderly patient receiving long-term care is not something that you do alone, ever! Caregivers absolutely need plentiful resources and help in order to provide good care. Chapter Nine lays out all of the forms of outside help available to you as a caregiver, from adult day care to hired companions, meal programs, and transportation.

While most elderly people very much want to stay in their own homes, it is not always possible, practical, or safe for that preference to be upheld. For many older people, a health crisis will precipitate the decision (by medical staff or caregivers) to move the patient into institutional living. Unfortunately decision-making in times of crisis is often rushed, reactive, and lacking in sound foundation. Chapter Ten addresses the questions and considerations you should sort out, ideally well in advance of that crisis, but even in the midst of it if necessary. You need to be able to accurately weigh your options when the time comes for your loved one to move out of his or her home. Chapter Eleven is devoted entirely to nursing homes, from making the decision to selecting a nursing home, crafting a plan of care, moving in, and getting adjusted.

Finally, Chapter Twelve: End of Life provides a holistic treatment of the topic of death and dying. There is no substitute for honest, clear information to help prepare caregivers for the painful reality of end-of-life care and the process of death itself. Thinking about the death of a loved one is never easy, and yet being informed and prepared is the greatest gift you can provide for yourself and the person you've loved and cared for until the end of life approaches.

While the bulk of this book is dedicated to seeing and accepting our current medical and long-term care systems for what they are, in order to make the best decisions and provide the best and most informed personal advocacy for your loved one, I urge you not to stop there. The final chapter of my book is dedicated to another type of advocacy—*political* advocacy. In Chapter Thirteen, I offer a road map for you and caregivers everywhere to join forces in a growing and powerful wave of political advocacy toward reforming our current system and creating a better one for the people we love, and, in the end, for all of us.

My inspiration for writing *The Good Caregiver* came from two sources. The first was my more than thirty years of studying aging and long-term care. The second (and ultimately more powerful) inspiration was the epiphany I experienced when I had to organize care for my own mother.[1] I soon learned that despite all my research, experience, and expertise, and despite my extensive network of colleagues across the country, I was not prepared to deal with what faced me. I learned that you cannot count on the system to do the right thing, but that instead you must be prepared to advocate for the right thing as much as possible. This book is meant to spare you from what I went through, and to give you a better chance of dealing with a system that, like the rest of our health care system, is broken.

---

1. Robert Kane and Joan West, *It Shouldn't Be This Way: The Future of Long-Term Care* (Nashville, 2005).

I have narrowed down a few guiding principles that underscore this whole book and everything in it. You should memorize these principles and revisit them every time you are faced with a new crisis or transition in caring for your loved one or yourself. Here they are, in no particular order:

Guiding Principles of Caregiving

- Caregiving can last a long time. Pace yourself. A baby boomer could be a caregiver for one or more family members for decades. Be a marathoner, not a sprinter.
- Long-term care can be expensive. Costs come both in dollars and in the toll it takes on everyone involved.
- Caregiving is hard work. Not everyone is cut out to be a caregiver.
- Families are central. Family members play a primary role in caregiving even after an older person is institutionalized. Sometimes they do it collectively. More often one or two family members rise to the challenge. When that happens, the rest of the family should do everything possible to support that effort. Absentee critics are not welcome.
- Set realistic expectations. Sometimes, expectations must be revised dramatically to fit reality. You might have to settle for less than you would expect if you were doing it all yourself, but you can't do it all by yourself all the time.
- Things change. Be prepared for the situation to shift and the concomitant demands to change as the frail person's condition changes.
- You must be the information clearinghouse. You cannot rely on the care system to remember things for the person getting the care.
- Be vigilant. Never assume that everything is being done as you expect.
- Choose your battles carefully. You cannot demand that everything be done to your standards, but you cannot ignore inadequate care or egregious assaults on quality of life.

- Professionals are only human. You are bound to encounter irrational responses from professionals.

That last principle might surprise you. Why should you encounter irrational responses from professionals? Shouldn't professionals be the ones you can always count on to be rational, calm, unbiased, and informed? Maybe, if they were not human. Professionals are drawn to doing what is comfortable and familiar, even when it is not necessarily what is best. Perhaps this would not be the case if our current medical system were not collapsing under the weight of underinsurance, overwhelming paperwork and regulation, and a seemingly endless number of "rules," some real and others imagined.

The situation is complicated by a perverse payment system that rewards doing more instead of doing better. Since health professionals *are* mere mortals, and the system *is* collapsing, one of the great challenges you are going face is trying to get medical staff to consider fresh ways to address problems in a system that's crumbling. Staff tend to see innovation as simply one more thing to do instead of a way to change or improve care. Families need to be advocates, and to encourage care that really focuses on the older person's needs instead of the needs of the staff or the "system." The good news is that there is increasing talk within long-term care circles about the need for this kind of patient-centered reform.

The Three Components of Quality Long-Term Care

Quality long-term care is complicated. It requires integrating three basic components: *personal assistance, housing*, and *medical care*. That may sound simple, but it is not. Hitting two out of three is not so hard, but getting the whole triad solidly in place is rarely achieved.

Personal Assistance

Personal assistance is not so tough if you have money or a devoted family. The best way is to hire someone who is devoted to providing the care. Paid caregivers work either on their own or in combination with family members to do the job. They may operate as independent contractors, working directly for a family, or they may be employees of an agency. But having the means to pay for care doesn't automatically mean you will get it. My sister and I struggled to organize care for my mother even while paying large sums for what we could cobble together. As for personal assistance in institutions, complaints in nursing homes are rampant, especially when it comes to close monitoring and intervention. One woman, trying to oversee care from a distance, described it this way: "The facility doesn't thoroughly or accurately assess Mom's abilities so that they don't have to provide a higher level of care—for example, to help her with the bathroom every two hours. Their argument is that they don't want to infringe on her dignity. But as a result, they're not providing safe care, and she frequently ends up wet or soiled."

Housing

Housing is also a matter of income: The richer you are, the nicer your house. But a nice house doesn't guarantee good care, either. Some people who live in plush surroundings may be neglected and even abused.[2] Fear of this very mistreatment can drive families to place older people in institutions in order to make sure the care is "well supervised." But there should never be a need to give up a more livable life in return for reliable care. In some situations it makes sense to house people close together to make the delivery of personal-care services more efficient. One wants to minimize travel time and use paid caregivers to treat as many people as possible. It is feasible to congregate people without putting them in institutions. But such congregation certainly does not mean those needing care should share

---

2. Remember the recent story of Brooke Astor, the heiress who suffered from terrible neglect.

a room with strangers. Congregate living does not automatically imply an institution. People live close to one another in apartments without giving up control of their lives. Institutional settings shouldn't automatically resort to institutional practices. Why shouldn't group living allow autonomy and choice? To some extent, college dorms manage this. Maybe we need more nursing homes where residents can order pizza and stay out late!

Good Medical Care

Good medical care is the hardest of the three components to achieve. Few doctors find frail older people interesting. Most doctors are very busy and many are enamored with technology. Besides, medical care is paid for as piecework, and doctors are under continuous pressure to see as many patients as possible. They don't have time for shooting the breeze with every patient. Time is money, and it's inefficient to give older patients the attention they crave and deserve. And older patients often suffer hearing problems and/or confusion, slowing things down even more. Very wealthy individuals can sometimes hire a personal clinician (ideally a board-certified geriatrician or a certified gerontological nurse practitioner) to provide "boutique" care (remember Howard Hughes?), but very few can afford that. And even when boutique care is an option, there's no guarantee that the provider will be particularly skilled with the problems of aging.

Finding a care system where the professionals in all three spheres—personal assistance, housing, and medical care—are competent is very hard. Most times the family has to become the glue that holds the three elements of care together.

Care, Money, and Compromise

For most people, long-term care requires compromises. Struggling to steer through emotionally and financially draining experiences, family members piece together the best care they can for their loved ones. Long-term care is at least as much an art as a science, and that makes it harder instead of easier. How do you determine in advance how much and what kind of care you will want and need later?

Good care costs money—lots of it—and no one wants to go overboard unnecessarily. But it is hard to determine just the right amount. We are used to thinking about needs as relatively objective, often based on a judgment made by an outside expert, like the Recommended Daily Value of calcium or calories. Wants, on the other hand, seem more subjective and tied up in our personal preferences and desires. In caring for the aging, those distinctions are less clear. No fixed rules can separate wants from needs or pinpoint the exact amount of care that is ideal or even appropriate. It's surprisingly easy to err in either direction.

Too much care can make a person unnecessarily dependent, while too little will cause useless and harmful struggle. For example, it is not ideal to stick every older person who walks with difficulty into a wheelchair. So designing nursing homes that reduce the distance residents need to walk for meals and other activities makes good sense. Rather than a single large dining room, smaller dining units on each wing might make dining easier and more pleasant, and keep residents more mobile. Besides, smaller dining rooms might help with hearing problems and facilitate a healthy social atmosphere.

On the other hand, a well-intentioned caregiving daughter whose elderly father was still employed despite a neurological condition encouraged her father to spend two hours and enormous energy dressing and showering himself each morning before paid caregivers came to take him to work. She made this arrangement to keep him from becoming unduly dependent for convenience and safety. It might have been better for the helpers to assist with this task, leaving her father to exercise independence at other times and in other ways.

Tough Decisions

Communication and cooperation are the essential ingredients to making rational choices at critical junctures. Without adequate communication and cooperation, most caregivers will settle for the most immediate solution, which in times of crisis will likely be a nursing home. As shadow extensions of the hospital, with many of the same faults and few of the benefits, nursing homes have largely outlived their usefulness. Nonetheless, representatives of these facilities tend to describe them as an extension of home in an effort to alleviate guilt for the family members. However, even a "nice" nursing home is not an extension of home.

Discussions about long-term care that ignore cost are fantasy. Many older people are reluctant to spend their own money on long-term care, preferring to retain a financial legacy they can pass on to their children and grandchildren. Even when the children (a strange term for people who are often in their sixties or seventies) insist that they neither need nor want the money, older people struggle to make do until a catastrophe robs them of choice in the matter. And then the pressure of making major decisions in the midst of a family and/or medical crisis too often leads to the older person entering a nursing home. Most people need a good system for making decisions under stress. We do not have "fire drills" for these challenges. The best most of us can hope for are reliable resources to help when the time comes.

Sometimes, caregivers base decisions on their own needs, as well as— or even instead of—the needs of the person receiving care. Adult children can't always afford to pay out-of-pocket for the care of an aging parent, and they may be understandably reluctant to mortgage their own children's futures. A full set of siblings might have the combined means to cover the cost of a parent's care, but even then, long-standing animosities or conflicting feelings about family roles can get in the way of moving ahead. Or families may fail to buy care that would make their own and their parent's life easier. Many families find it hard to seek help, thinking they should be able to do it themselves. But caregiving can be taxing. Not everyone is cut out for the sacrifices entailed (remember that you can find in Chapter One the guidelines of caregiving and a personal assessment for families to gauge their capacity to give care). It is important to remember that such decisions are not cast in stone; they need to be reexamined periodically as the realities become more apparent and situations change.

Advocacy Toward a Better Future

In an immediate sense, this book is intended to help you navigate the caregiving system as it currently exists. You cannot serve yourself or your loved one without understanding and accepting the real-life options you will face, even if those options are imperfect. But in the long run, we should all be advocating for a better system of care for elderly adults. It should not be necessary to share multiperson rooms with strangers, adhering to routines created for the convenience of staff, and meanwhile be deprived of the amenities that make life interesting and enjoyable. It should be feasible in this day and age to get personal care in a setting where a person can still lead a meaningful life and retain a sense of personhood and dignity.

Better Models for Community Living

Several model programs already exist for both institutional and community settings that work much better to meet the needs of the elderly. For example, assisted-living facilities evolved as a direct response to the way nursing homes force residents to live. Assisted-living environments address residents first and foremost as tenants, providing living space that residents can call their own. Residents maintain control over their own living quarters, including who comes into them; and they remain in charge of their basic daily routines. But as the number and diversity of assisted-living facilities grew, regulatory problems sprang up. Critics cried foul, saying that if assisted living cared for residents who would otherwise be in nursing homes, then the same standards should apply to both. However, supporters of assisted living countered that the same regulations would simply convert assisted-living facilities into nursing homes. The debate continues to this day.

Meanwhile, some nursing home models are trying to address living arrangement problems. Newer designs are breaking nursing home institutions into smaller "neighborhoods" or "households" with more consistent staffing and greater autonomy. Residents are encouraged to become more actively involved in daily activities, including food preparation, but regulations still pose barriers. For example, some fear that residents might be exploited or coerced into doing work that should be done by staff.

But all of this matters little for most of those navigating the long-term care system for loved ones right now. While the arguments rage on, neither assisted living nor more "evolved" nursing homes are available to the vast majority of those needing and wanting options. Easy access to quality choices in elder care will require major shifts politically, economically, medically, and individually.

A Call to Action

We need massive citizen demand for reform. Maybe the time has arrived for this. After all, things won't get any easier in the coming decades. Our population is aging, and spending on long-term care for the elderly is projected to more than double over the next thirty years. Politicians, insurance companies, and health care providers need to come together soon. The over-eighty-five-year-old population is the fastest growing segment of our population, and 50 percent of the "oldest old" need assistance in daily functioning. No politician is speaking out about this, and meanwhile, as pointed out by Peter Strauss, chairman of the Elder Care Task Force of the New York Business Group, the costs of caring for these older persons is impoverishing middle-income Americans. For those interested in learning more about joining the reform effort, the last chapter of this book will give you a good start on the path of informed advocacy for a more humane system.

One

Becoming a Caregiver

My mom died of Alzheimer's disease, and she and my dad, who also needed care, spent around half a million dollars over eight years. I have nothing like that to rely on—and never will.

—Liz Taylor, *Aging Deliberately* columnist

A CAREGIVER'S STORY

My mother is ninety-one, still in her own home. But without my visiting four or five times a week, she couldn't do that. Whatever I do for her to try to make life easier, more interesting, or more fun, it's never right. I am doing my best to make her latter days peaceful and worry-free, and I forgive a lot and bite my tongue constantly. I'm fifty-nine, a recently retired health care provider, and the only daughter. Since my retirement, my brothers and their wives must have clapped their hands and clearly think it's all down to me now, and how very convenient for them. My husband is supportive of me but sees how heavy-hearted I am these days. He and I wonder if our retirement will ever be ours to enjoy. I'll continue to do what I can for my mother, I love her dearly. I don't expect effusive thanks from Mom for anything I do, I just wish she wouldn't whine and moan and complain that the "boys" would have done it so much better! Sometimes, in an effort to forget and to comfort myself, I drink too much (I'm ashamed and I know how bad that is for my health), and then I get up the next day and go see Mother, take her shopping, have coffee/lunch with her, take her home, and apologize in response to her critical comments about how brief was my stay. Today was

(*story continued*)

a bad day and I have found myself on the verge of tears all day, yet trying to act cheerful-ish and come home with a smile on my face. Think carefully, all those who are highly critical of caregivers who give their all, with no pay, often no thanks, often with an expectation by family, society, and the medical profession, that the daughters will sacrifice everything—after all, it's what daughters do, isn't it? We're growing older, too, in a world that has the science to ensure that our elderly parents live even longer.

—CAREGIVING DAUGHTER

M ost people do not plan to be caregivers. They are thrust into the role by fate and circumstances. Sometimes it is easy to predict who will assume that role; they have been caring for someone all their lives, but sometimes the choice is quite unexpected and the person chosen is all the more unprepared for the role.

Deciding who should become the primary caregiver requires an open discussion within the family. Not all families are prepared to have that discussion. A lot of old family dynamics may come into play. It is a time for honest introspection. Preferences certainly play a role. Not everyone is cut out to be a caregiver, either by temperament or by circumstances. Some people have other great responsibilities. Some opt to make major life changes in order to take on a new caregiving role.

My sister and I became caregivers when my mother suffered a stroke. From that day until my mother died three years later, my sister was in constant attendance. My mother spent most of her last years in assisted living, where my sister visited her almost every day. I had the much easier role as the outside expert and support person. My sister and I talked most nights on the phone and I visited my sister and mother periodically. Fortunately, we agreed on virtually every aspect of our mother's care and options.

When it became clear early on that my mother could not live on her own, we decided she had to live near one of us. In many ways we could have gotten cheaper, perhaps better care for her in Minneapolis than on Long Island, but there was no question that my sister would be the more devoted caregiver. Moreover, my sister would have felt very frustrated if my mother came to Minneapolis. Caregiving took a great toll on my sister, but she also found it very rewarding. Even though my mother was in assisted living, my sister saw her constantly, handling all of Mom's doctor visits, as well as other outings for shopping and dining in restaurants. She had a strong sense of needing to be there and would have felt very guilty doing anything less.

A TOTAL COMMITMENT

Caregiving is a *total* commitment. It ends up being your life. You never feel like you do enough. It is important to think of yourself and your health and of others who love you. When I began to develop heart problems and strained my abdomen when lifting my mother after a fall, I reevaluated the situation and realized it was time for professionals to begin providing care for my mother.

I have no regrets for doing that. I enjoyed the time I was able to spend with my mother as long as I was physically and mentally able. But when you are in this type of situation it's very important to realize that it is a difficult thing to do and it's okay to reevaluate the circumstances and make a conscious decision about not being able to do it anymore.

—SANDY, CAREGIVING DAUGHTER

If you are a family member who just woke up to find yourself in the role of caregiver to your parent or other relative, you are not alone. Family members provide the vast majority of long-term care, typically in their own or the older person's own private home. Some say that as much as 95 percent of all long-term care gets provided in this way, by what the system refers to as "informal caregivers." Although men certainly provide some "informal care,"[3] that phrase is basically a euphemism

---

3. See William Wharton's fictionalized account of caring for his father, *Dad* (New York: Knopf, 1981).

that usually refers to women—wives, daughters, and daughters-in-law. Remarriage and domestic-partner arrangements can create some unusual circumstances as well, and former daughters-in-law and even ex-wives may become unexpected caregivers at times.

Despite strong feelings of obligation and social pressure, it can be a great mistake to undertake caregiving if you are ill suited or ill prepared. Making the commitment deserves serious consideration. Caregivers have been shown to have more physical and mental illness than those who do not give such care. One element of this decision-making should involve an honest self-assessment. The Minnesota Family Self-Assessment Test offers a simple set of questions that will help you set off on this journey. Answer the questions and review your answers to get some insights into your situation. Discuss your answers with those who will also be affected by your caregiving decision: your spouse, your siblings, perhaps your children.

The Minnesota Family Self-Assessment Test

Each potential caregiver should ask him/herself the following questions:

	Questions	Yes	No
1.	Am I physically able to provide the needed assistance? (Could I continue doing this work for weeks? Months? Years? Do I have physical limitations for the work involved?)		
2.	Do my skills fit the profile of the tasks that need to be done?		
3.	Am I prepared to perform intimate caregiving chores like bathing and helping with toileting?		
4.	Think about the kinds of help your relative needs. Do I have the temperament to be a caregiver for a sustained period? (Will I become easily upset and angry? Am I able to stay calm and treat family members with patience and kindness even when I feel tired and overworked with the responsibilities of being a caregiver?)		
5.	Can I free my schedule to be available when needed? (Can I free my schedule to be available at a moment's notice or for extended periods of time? Is my schedule flexible enough to provide help whenever needed?)		

	Questions	Yes	No
6.	Can I afford to reduce or stop working? (Do I need to continue to work for pay to meet the current or future or financial needs for myself or my family?)		
7.	Am I willing to reduce or neglect other obligations in order to give the care needed? (Do I have any roles or responsibilities that cannot be neglected?)		
8.	Am I free of other people who already depend on my help (e.g., children, relatives)?		
9.	Will giving care unduly stress other family relationships, e.g., with my spouse or other family members?		
Caregiver Readiness Total (number of "yes" answers in items 1–9)			
10.	Can I protect myself from getting so involved that I never take a break or get help? (Am I willing to ask for help if I need it? Is there help readily available for respite care? Do I have a list of contacts to ask for help when I need a break?)		
11.	Would I be willing to purchase care to supplement the care I can give? (Do I have the financial resources to purchase supplemental care? Would I be willing to pay someone to help me provide the care that is needed?)		
12.	Do the people around me support me in my decision? (Are they willing to share in some of the responsibilities? Do the important people in my life know about the responsibilities I am taking as a caregiver? Do they agree with my taking that role?)		
Caregiver Protection Total (number of "yes" answers in items 10–12)			
13.	Will giving care change my relationship with the older person?		
14.	If I am unable to provide direct care, do I have the adequate financial resources to provide for the type of care that is needed?		

Interpreting Your Responses to the Self-Assessment

This is not a quiz; there are no right or wrong answers. It is a self-diagnostic tool, designed to spur you to insights. Look at the pattern of your responses and decide if you are prepared to undertake the caregiver role. The first nine items address issues that should be answered affirmatively if you are ready to take on caregiving. If you cannot say "yes" to at least six, you should think carefully about taking on the caregiver role. In some cases even one question can be a deal breaker. Items 10 to 12 address ways of getting support to maintain caregiving. You should have some of those if you are going to succeed. The last two items are things to think about; they may not directly affect your decision, but they will influence your caregiving experience. You may not be ready to give a definite yes/no answer to some questions. In those cases, they should serve as prompts for areas where you need to learn more, or discuss these topics with family and others.

Informal Care: The Essential and Instrumental Activities of Daily Living

Much of informal caregiving is day-to-day assistance and supervision with routine tasks that were once independent: eating, dressing, using the bathroom, moving from bed to chair. These are essential activities of daily living, or ADLs. More complex tasks such as cooking, shopping, cleaning, using the telephone, laundering, banking, and negotiating transportation are called instrumental activities of daily living, or IADLs. Being independent means being able to manage essential and instrumental activities. The inability to perform these tasks alone is typically the trigger for a family's beginning to consider institutional living arrangements for their loved one.

Not surprisingly, couples do better than older people who live on their own when it comes to the ADLs. Spouses have frequently developed instinctive coping mechanisms that are difficult to describe. Their behavior can look dysfunctional to others, but it is effective. Each member of the couple has a role. Children may wonder how their parents manage, but they do. Because most chronic problems come on slowly, almost without anyone being aware, the coping mechanisms also tend to evolve in a similarly organic and unspoken process. But what comes naturally to a spouse is often more difficult for other caregivers. In many cases, spouses have been doing some assistive tasks before the onset of dependency. Certainly tasks like cooking and laundry are familiar household tasks. Spouses usually take on caregiving tasks subtly. In the early stages it may be hard to tell what is done as part of normal family life and what is caregiving.

Effective help with daily tasks makes it possible for a frail older person to survive and thrive. Help can involve providing hands-on assistance with personal care or managing finances, shopping, cooking, transportation, or even social support. It may be as simple as lending an arm, making a phone

DON'T GO IT ALONE

Find out about the local resources and talk to people who are using these services. There are aging services resource centers or Area Agencies on Aging in every county in every state. They have free telephone consultants who can help you find out about local resources for everyday needs, such as transportation, home-delivered meals, homemaker services, yard work, home repair, and so on. You will want to get a list and then check them out. Always try to meet them outside of your home and preferably with a local aging services advocate guiding you with what questions to ask and how the service is set up. Do your homework and follow your gut. Do not sign a contract with anyone—at least not until you have had a trial run and have had good results. If it is a paid service, go online to the state website and see what kind of rating or certification the organization has. Check with the Better Business Bureau. Talk to as many people as you can in terms of what works well for people in the situation you are in and what does not. There are also national websites for help. For the first visit, be there when the service provider shows up and be attentive to the service they provide. If you are unhappy, tell them. My mother did not want a paid home care agency, both because of expense and because of her feelings of vulnerability about "strangers" coming into her home. But she did accept the installation of grab bars in her shower and bathroom, new railings at all entrances, new railings on both sides of her stairwell, walkers, an "electric recliner" chair, and paid yard work help.

—DEB PAONE, CAREGIVING DAUGHTER

call, or charting a path; or it may prove more demanding, such as pushing a wheelchair. Some caregivers will need to master technical nursing skills, like managing a ventilator or giving injections. And major conflicts about autonomy can crop up. For example, older persons who need assistance with shopping still want a major voice in what's purchased. An adult child trying to be sure that Mom gets nutritious food may infuriate a woman who wants to decide for herself whether to eat white bread or wheat.

Speaking of eating, it can be a touchy subject for older people whose faulty vision and tremors interfere with neatness at mealtimes. You may feel embarrassed by your parent's sloppy eating habits, and be reluctant to take her to restaurants. But your parent may be oblivious to these lapses. Get over it. So what if strangers take umbrage. It is a shame to deprive Mom or Dad of an enjoyable experience for the sake of appearances alone.

Many older people cope with restrictions in physical and mental functioning by developing fixed routines and habits that can seem irrational and irksome for caregivers. But it is probably not worth the fight. Better to step back and admire how well rather than how poorly the older person copes with her realities.

When Care Feels Taboo

Some informal caregiving can be very intimate and personal. You may find yourself doing things for your parent that violate long-held taboos. For example, sons do not look at the naked bodies of their mothers', nor daughters at their fathers'. But you cannot help your parent bathe or dress without taking her clothes off. Washing genital areas or helping your parent use the bathroom can seem even more invasive. But human beings are remarkably resilient. It is surprising how rapidly you both can adapt to new standards for behavior when the most basic personal needs are at stake.

I recall clearly being with my mother in the hospital on a day when the nurses seemed totally preoccupied with everyone else and had no time for her. Even though I am a doctor and am used to examining women, I felt very uncomfortable taking my mother to the bathroom and having to help her dress and undress. Her complete lack of concern made it easier to forget that my mother was a very private person, but it was disconcerting nonetheless.

The Overcaring Trap

Beware of overcaring. It is always faster and easier to do things for a frail older person than to work with them to do tasks themselves. Too much care can have a perverse effect. If you take over too much of what your parent can do for herself, you'll encourage unnecessary dependence. Compassion and sincere desire to help make it is easy to fall into this trap. Sometimes family members rush to do tasks because the older person does them so slowly that it causes frustration and impatience. You need to steel yourself against this and resist the urge to do too much. Better to encourage and assist your parent to do for herself whenever possible. The lasting benefits are well worth the extra effort.

It is very easy to fall into this trap. Paid caregivers do it all the time, especially when they have multiple clients to care for. Given a work quota and production expectations, nursing aides are strongly tempted to do what is most expedient. Frail older people are often slow and sloppy. They may perseverate over decisions, and make bad ones. We are in a hurry and want the job done right. But this is narrow, short-term thinking. Older persons may have little sense of time and nothing to fill it with. It may be better for all to let them retain control of elements of their lives. What are you going to do with all the time you saved if you still have to entertain them? Who is really offended if their clothes don't quite match?

Care Management

Family caregivers may also need to serve as care managers. You will quickly discover that you know more about what is going on than anyone else, including all those professionals you expect to know. That means you have to be very organized. You will probably need to coordinate care to ensure that one doctor knows what other doctors have done. You cannot rely on the doctors to know that. You must aggressively tell them what their colleagues have done and prescribed. To do that you will need to maintain up-to-date lists of diagnoses, treatments, and medications. And you'll have to maintain the full and current roster of doctors providing care for your parent (including phone numbers). You will need a good system for keeping track of medications prescribed to avoid duplications and assure that medication lists are current. Equally challenging is scheduling appointments and tests, and making sure Mom or Dad gets to the appointed place at the appointed hour (if only to then wait to be seen).

Role Reversal

Parental aging can bring on gradual transitions in family roles even before an older person becomes disabled. Roles become subtly reversed. Children begin advising their parents, while parents look to their children for guidance and approval. I remember exactly when this happened

Calling a doctor's office can be a trying experience for someone who is cognitively intact and able to hear perfectly. You get recorded messages and are put on hold. Imagine what it is like for someone who has compromised hearing or vision. It is wise for a family member to keep track of all the logistics. My brother-in-law was the primary caregiver for his father. He kept meticulous records of every doctor, dentist, and other health professional, including contact information and the name of the receptionist. He prepared a daily calendar of all medications and appointments.

for me. About a year after my father died, my mother invited my wife and me to meet her new boyfriend. The boyfriend (in his late sixties) came to the door in white slacks and a blazer (as if he were dressed for the prom) and I sat across from him waiting for my mother and my wife to get dressed. It was like a scene from a Norman Rockwell painting. He sat with his hands folded in his lap, and it was all I could do to keep from asking about school. My wife and I were clearly the chaperones that night. My role was to grant approval for my mother's choice.

Balancing Protection with Respect

But sometimes the adult kids start offering advice before it's requested, especially when they worry about their parents' safety. And here is where it is clear that role reversal is a mixed analogy. Parents are morally and legally responsible for their young children. But adult children of older parents have much more limited roles, unless they have actually been appointed as legal guardians of their parents. They act out of concern, and there may be genuine need for their involvement, but they have to respect the wishes of the elders as much as possible. The younger generation tends to be more cautious than their parents. They want their parents to be protected at all costs, but this concern over safety robs older persons of their autonomy and disrupts their lifestyles.

There is a temptation to view frail older persons as equivalent to children, with the biological children taking on parental roles. This is a mistake. While some roles and responsibilities may shift, older parents are not children. They have a history. They have raised you and deserve to be treated as adults as long as possible, even if they are unable to remain the dominant adult.

When Parents Won't Plan

At the other extreme, caregivers can suffer the consequences of their older parents' poor decisions. What happens when your parents avoid making plans for getting older, refuse to move near family, and a crisis ensues? The adult children are left with the fallout, much of which could have been prevented or diminished had some plans been made in advance. In one example from a colleague, an eighty-five-year-old woman was providing care in her own home to her ninety-year-old husband, who suffered dementia and blindness. There were no plans for the husband's likely decline. The five adult children were kept out of the decision-making loop. Eventually, when one child developed colon cancer and could no longer make the trip to visit her parents, the parents moved, with great reluctance. On their own, they purchased an apartment that turned out to be an ill-advised investment. Within a year, the wife/caregiver died after a trajectory of slow decline and poor medical care. The stresses and conflicts prior to her death reached such a pitch that a restraining order was even put into place against one of the daughters. The elderly couple's home did not sell, nor did the apartment, leaving a financial mess that took a long time to be sorted out by the adult children.

Siblings Sharing Caring

Ideally, the burden of care gets spread out among siblings, even if one sibling takes the bulk of responsibility. But many families are in no condition to divvy up responsibilities so easily. Families are geographically dispersed. Siblings have old roles and rivalries. Some family members are better off paying for professional care than providing it in person. Inevitably, the uneven distribution of work tears open long-standing family issues. Caregiving crises can arise. One sibling becomes the dominant caregiver, but the others feel free to criticize the care given. Sometimes, the conflicts can only be resolved with the help of family therapy. If you and your siblings are struggling initially over the division of responsibility and decision-making about caregiving, it may help to begin with seeking the assistance of a counselor or therapist early on, to act as a neutral but skilled facilitator of your discussions.

When Family Members Disagree

No aging-related decision is easy. Risk and privacy have to be balanced against safety and the stress of change. Different family members may have wildly out-of-sync views on the same matter. Caught in the middle, an aging parent can be treated like an inanimate object for whom plans are made, instead of a central figure in the decision-making. Older persons need to be included as primary players in deciding their fate, but conflicts will inevitably arise. What happens when the older person insists she can remain at home when everyone else believes it is far too risky? There is no simple answer. In the end one's tolerance for risk and respect for an older person's autonomy must be balanced. The key issue is actually talking about these things. All too often the subject is avoided and family members attempt to hoodwink the older person (presumably in their best interest). Involving the older person is obviously much more complex when she is suffering from dementia.

Often, even though the bulk of day-to-day caregiving is shouldered by a single family member, the rest of the family chimes in freely with complaints or concerns, or even accuses the primary caregiver of neglect. In a crisis, however, families as a whole often do and should share the caregiving burden, taking their lead from the primary caregiver. A relative who has played no role in caregiving may feel a need to become actively involved in decision-making around a crisis point.

When Dementia Complicates Decisions

When dementia is involved, caregiving often requires twenty-four-hour supervision. Most family members are insecure about leaving a person with even minimally advanced dementia alone for fear she will create a hazardous situation. Experience has shown that this level of concern is often excessive. The line between neglect and encouraging autonomy may be hard to draw with confidence. Just as with raising children there are dangers in being too protective or too laissez-faire, so dementia presents questions about how much risk can be tolerated. Many persons with severe dementia are able to live on their own with only periodic visits each day to make sure that they are eating and staying clean. Obviously, you have to take steps in these cases to make sure that the environment is safe. For example, stoves might need to be disconnected, water temperatures lowered, throw rugs removed, and lighting improved; and steps, bathtubs, and showers must have grab bars professionally installed. People with impaired cognition may also be victimized by various types of solicitors. They make an easy mark for telemarketers, and can be too easily influenced by those close to them into giving away money or making poor investments. It is important to monitor their bank accounts and their checkbooks.

It Can Be Done: Safe Caregiving and Dementia

Families worry a great deal about persons with dementia living on their own and potentially wandering off and getting into difficulty. The extent of this concern should vary with the circumstances. Obviously you do not want a demented person wandering off in the middle of a Minnesota winter and dying of hypothermia. And no one is comfortable with a person wandering unaware in a major metropolitan area. But many environments can support wandering.

In small towns, neighbors often come to recognize the person with dementia and can either bring him home or contact the police, who are usually quite supportive. We visited a program in Adelaide, Australia (admittedly a mild climate), that cared for persons with Alzheimer's disease living on their own in their own homes. They were visited daily to be sure they were eating and performing basic tasks, but otherwise left largely to their own devices. Police and other groups were alerted to look out for these people and return them to their homes if they were found outside. The proponents of this program argued that much of the stress in caring for such people comes from conflict with caregivers. If there are no caregivers around for much of the time, there are fewer rage reactions and behavior problems. There are no systematic studies of such programs, but they open up some interesting possibilities. The Alzheimer's Association has developed a program called Safe Return, which provides ID products and an enrollment procedure that makes it easier to identify someone who has wandered off. (Web resources in the appendix at the end of the book provide more information.)

Technology may help families feel more comfortable with the idea of frail older people living on their own. A variety of devices allow an older person to summon help. Simple button-activated devices can make phone calls, and remote microphones can be worn around the neck or as a bracelet.

When Money Matters Cause Problems

Managing money is particularly likely to cause problems. Older people may not want their children to know their financial status. Disclosing our money matters is a major invasion of privacy. People are more willing to tell you their weight or their age than their incomes or credit scores. In many cases, as an older person becomes more confused and unable to manage personal finances, it becomes necessary to make an adult child a cosignatory with durable power of attorney to withdraw funds from the elder person's bank account. This position carries great responsibility. The caregiver must always keep the older person's interests paramount. But this is easier said than done. The cosignator likely will struggle at some point, asking whether it is in the older person's best interest to preserve assets or spend her money for care. As noted above, adult children may be more anxious to purchase care than their aging parents, who may prefer to "make do." On the other hand, some children may have a strong need for their inheritance and may be reluctant to see it spent on their parents' care.

When Guardianship Is Needed

The extreme case is guardianship or conservatorship. In some cases it may be necessary to literally wrest control of an older person's decision-making about financial matters and even his or her own care. This requires a legal procedure whereby the person is adjudicated as incompetent to manage his own affairs and someone is appointed as guardian. This guardian may be a family member or someone hired (often at considerable cost) to perform the task. The guardian should be truly disinterested, that is, have nothing personal to gain from the decisions made. Obviously a relative waiting for a large inheritance may not make the best guardian. It is a position of great power and responsibility. Once guardianship has been assigned it is hard to revoke. It is thus not something to be entered into lightly. Guardianships can go dreadfully wrong. Guardians may have strong feelings about safety, for example, and rely unnecessarily on institutionalization. Substantial portions of an older person's remaining resources may go to paying the guardian.

A CAUTIONARY TALE

Once guardianship has been initiated it may be hard to undo. A middle-aged Minnesota woman, incapacitated by malnutrition and a prolonged bout of heavy drinking, was taken to a nearby hospital. When her mental condition failed to improve over a month's time, the state courts appointed a guardian, who determined that she needed to be cared for in a nursing home. She has been sober and well fed for a year. Although she has dramatically improved to the point where she can eat, dress herself, and use the bathroom without assistance, she still lives in the nursing home. Her neurologist pronounced her healthy enough to move back home. However, her court-appointed professional guardian has determined she is not fit to leave. The more she has tried to take control of her life, the harder the system has fought to keep her a ward of the state.

—JAMES ELI SHIFFER, *MINNEAPOLIS STAR TRIBUNE*, AUGUST 26, 2009

Institutional Care: A Different Facet of Caregiving

If and when institutional or residential care is the best or only option, your caregiving does not end. When an older person enters an assisted-living facility, nursing home, or other group-living arrangement, you must remain eternally vigilant to be sure that needed care is provided and no compromising events occur. But you must also advocate to promote a good quality of life. In assisted living, family will be expected to provide their relative with needed supplies, arrange appointments, and so on. By contrast, in nursing homes family may be discouraged from playing an active role. In both settings, residents need to be engaged. Social support is also crucially important. Frequent visiting is vital, even if it's painful. As older people adapt to life in institutional settings, their interests in other things tend to narrow. Sometimes this narrowing may be induced if the older person is excluded from family news and gossip. It becomes harder to engage them in conversation. But whatever you do, do not give up. Continue to visit and to do whatever possible to engage your parent however you can. Try outings. They will be appreciated and can be therapeutic. Meals in restaurants are also a treat, and a welcome break from the institutional menu, no matter how excellent the kitchen and varied the offerings.

But taking a frail parent out to eat can be a challenge. Whenever I came to visit my mother I took her out to a Chinese restaurant (her favorite food). As her disease progressed she had more trouble eating, especially eating neatly. She would create a penumbra of food all around her (and on her), but she was oblivious to the mess. Although it may have had some modest negative effect on her fellow diners, and certainly made more work for the waitstaff, I judged it a worthwhile event. I compensated by tipping generously.

My enthusiasm for taking my mother out finally met its Waterloo. I kept telling my sister that it was still possible to take our mother out to restaurants and promised to show her when I next visited. My sister, my brother-in-law, and I went to see my mother and bundled her into a wheelchair to get her to the car to go out for a pizza lunch. (Pizza is a great food for people who eat with their hands.) It was a bit of work, but we managed to get her into the car. We drove to the restaurant and then proceeded to get her out of the car and into the wheelchair. She offered little assistance and was basically dead weight. We could not pull her out of the seat without hurting her. So my brother-in-law slid into the other side of the backseat to push while I pulled and pivoted her into the wheelchair. We almost made it, but ultimately she collapsed back onto him. It was hilarious but sad. We burst out laughing, bundled her back into the car, and drove back to the assisted living, where we brought in a pizza, which we ate in some private dining space.

When your parent gets too frail to go out, you can bring in favorite foods. Sometimes this can cause an uproar with staff, if your goodies violate dietary orders. Sometimes you can convince staff to make an exception or turn a blind eye, especially if you organize the eating in your parent's private room or some space out of public view. Sometimes you can bribe the staff by providing treats for them as well.

Advocacy

Advocacy is crucial to your older person getting good care in an institution. Residents with advocates get better care than those without them. Advocacy is also critical to getting good care from health professionals and organizations. But being an effective advocate is hard. It is a little like the Kenny Rogers song about the gambler: You have to know when to hold and when to fold. Advocacy includes investigating and weighing evidence from various sources. It may be difficult to know how to react when your parent says she is being abused or mistreated by the nursing home staff. Is this a hallucination or might it be real? It is often hard to know. Verifying complaints is tricky. Still, you have to take the statements seriously. A recurring grievance of nursing home residents is that staff do not arrive

VISITING AS AN OFFERING, NOT AN OBLIGATION

My mother spent three and a half years in a nursing home as a result of Alzheimer's disease. At that time, I was working and raising a son, so I had to place her under institutional care. I did, however, spend one to two hours with her every evening, getting her ready for bed. The nursing home was so understaffed that her comfort needs were not being met.

I made these daily visits, not as an obligation, but as an offering. I would not allow my mother to become victimized by her disease, isolated from society, forgotten, or given substandard care. Not that most of the nursing home staff wasn't caring—it's just that the organizational structure and lack of funding resulted in difficult working conditions.

I also felt that the end of life is a time of spiritual connections. As the Alzheimer's symptoms increased, my mother spent more time in "conversation" with beings that I could not see or hear. As my mother gazed upward, and shifted her gaze as though addressing different people, she would talk in clear sentences, although by now she had stopped communicating verbally with the rest of us.

There was much to weep about during my mother's last three and a half years. But despite all the difficulties, the inner connection between us survived. What my mother taught me was the power of love.

—ELANNE PALCICH, CAREGIVING DAUGHTER

soon enough for toileting needs. Fear of accidents caused by having to wait too long can discourage older residents from drinking enough liquids. And soiling accidents lead to other problems, like bedsores, which emerge easily if the skin is not kept clean and dry. But staff who weather these complaints continuously can feel as if they cannot possibly do enough to keep the resident's family satisfied.

Families need to remember that they always have the option of leaving. If you cannot get satisfactory care, you should move your relative to another facility, or even take her home for a while. The big problem is inertia. Once you relocate an older relative, it takes a lot of effort to make a change, even when one is indicated.

LESSONS FOR BEING A GOOD ADVOCATE

Understand that you are becoming your parent's advocate, but he or she still is in the driver's seat. There is a delicate dance between advocating and taking over. I had to bite the inside of my cheek sometimes not to say something when my mother was choosing a course of action that was her right to decide even though I did not agree. The primary example was her decision to wait for one year before trying chemotherapy. She asked my opinion once, I gave it, and then she made her decision. After that, my job was to be there for her. In the early stages it was clear that she could make her own decisions and had clear thinking. In mid- to later stages I saw more decisions being made out of denial or hope rather than rational thinking, but if they did not endanger her and there was a way to accommodate without extensive difficulty, then my role was to help her continue to be in control of her life.

There are three key pieces to being a good advocate. First, you have to be there—in the room—when things are happening. Second, you have to know what your loved one would prefer, and third, you have to be able to make a clear-headed, reasonable suggestion in your nicest voice possible while still making it clear that you are speaking on the patient's/person's behalf to make clear his or her preferences. Suggested phrases to use are "We are hoping you could find a way to accommodate _____ (fill in name) by doing or arranging for _____ (fill in activity or thing that is needed) because it would help him/her to adapt to this latest issue. Can you help us with that?" Another piece of advocacy is offering information that is important to the person you are trying to get to make a change—for example: "The last time my mother tried this medicine she had real stomach issues and could not eat. Since we are trying to have her gain weight, do you think there is something else that we could do to counteract that or is there another less potent drug or dose that would be therapeutic?"

—DEB PAONE, CAREGIVING DAUGHTER

The 80/20 Rule

Advocating for a frail older person is tricky. Concerned and vigilant family members may observe many mistakes and oversights, but you have to choose your battles wisely. Challenging every infraction can create endless friction and alienate the staff beyond repair. The squeaky wheel may get the grease, but the constantly squeaking wheel eventually gets ignored. Worse yet, if you're seen as a nag, you might cause the staff to be even less attentive to your relative as an act of retaliation. Staff are only human, and human nature means that there might be some negative fall-out because of your constant complaining. That is enough reason to give pause before crusading on every minor issue. Save your ammunition for when it counts. And sometimes it does.

While you have to use judgment and restraint, never let fear send you shrinking from challenging the system when something important is compromised or overlooked. Institutions can be dangerous places. Problems may go unheeded. Mistakes get made, sometimes serious ones. Having an advocate is crucial to a successful stay in an institution, even one that seeks to provide active and caring support. Recently, a number of successful lawsuits have been filed against nursing homes for inadequate care. But be careful. Legal action should be reserved for only those instances when you believe grievous neglect has occurred and all other remedies have failed.

One colleague has recommended the 80/20 rule. Try to compliment the nursing home staff at least four times as often as you raise complaints. Staff members respond well to praise and are grateful when they sense that families appreciate their efforts. Compliments validate positive behaviors and build trust. Then, your constructive criticism may be more easily accepted. Most institutions don't allow you to tip staff, for fear it would literally buy better care for bigger tips. But many homes will allow families to bring in small treats for the staff. If so, do not hesitate to celebrate this way whenever your mom or dad has a good response to care. One colleague told me that it never hurts to bring treats for the staff when your loved one does well. He said, "I used to do that when my aunt had a good day or turned a corner after an illness. It really helped—especially since these people earn so little and work double shifts frequently. Cakes or cases of popcorn from Costco earned a lot of brownie points for me."

Fast Help for Serious Problems

If you do encounter a serious care problem or feel there has been neglect or abuse, seek help immediately. Your first response should probably be to contact the Nursing Home Ombudsman, whose contact information should be posted in a very obvious and prominent location, usually next to a public or pay telephone. There is an Ombudsman office in every state. You may want to consult the National Citizens' Coalition for Nursing Home Reform's *Nursing Homes: Getting Good Care There*. It includes valuable instruction on how to complain effectively to nursing home administrators about the care.

Family Councils

Many nursing homes have councils where family members can meet with staff to voice concerns and help develop care plans. Family councils provide a powerful forum for voicing problems as well as praising good care. It is worth the time to be part of them. Woody Allen is quoted as saying that 80 percent of success is showing up. By being involved as much as possible, through visiting often and attending conferences, you go a long way toward increasing the quality of care for your loved one and others.

Avoiding Caregiver Burnout

It goes by a lot of names: caregiver burnout, compassion fatigue, but it is a very real threat. If you plan on caring for someone for an extended period of time, you should develop a plan to avoid caregiver burnout. Caregiving is a hard job. There is no nine-to-five schedule, and you are always on call. You never feel like you are doing enough. The more committed you are, the less you are satisfied with your performance. This commitment takes a toll. You may not be aware of it, but people around you will see it. In order to make it through day after day of this demanding schedule, you may adopt the belief that no one can take your place.

This is completely understandable. But, obviously, this attitude makes it very hard for you to take a break. It is not only egotistical; it may be more selfish than selfless. A worn-out caregiver cannot give very good care. The FAA makes pilots take rest periods to refresh themselves to prevent plane crashes. Caregivers need to prevent care crashes. Everyone needs some time away from such a stressful task. Caregiver burnout ultimately harms both the caregiver and the patient. More information on caregiver burnout and respite care is provided in Chapters Four and Nine.

Things Change

The path of caregiving is not straight. There will be many ups and downs. The condition of the care recipient will change over time and those changes will have implications for the caregiving role. Most of the changes, alas, involve worsening conditions and concomitant added burdens. These may come in the form of more actual help or a deterioration in behavior that means more coping and adapting. Sometimes these changes are acute—for example, the older person falls and breaks a hip—but often they occur subtly. You look up one day and realize that you are doing a lot more than you bargained for.

Human beings are remarkably adaptable. We cope with change. But we also have breaking points. It is important to periodically reassess the caregiving demands you face and decide if they are impinging too much on your life.

Sometimes the caregiving crisis comes not from the added burden of new problems but from a change in circumstances. Other demands on you increase. Other people in the immediate family need more support or assistance. These are moments when you need to reevaluate the sustainability of your caregiving. Do not shrink from reality. You will do no one a favor by working yourself to death or depression.

The response need not be all or none. The best solution may be to get more help—from family or by purchasing it.

Planning for the Future

Planning for long-term care is hard but necessary and worth the effort. As you enter into the planning process, it helps to be realistic, and to recognize that while realistic may seem negative, realism actually helps avoid more heartbreak than the lack of preparation created through false hopes and denial. There are no easy long-term care decisions. Sadly, no matter what you decide to do, you will probably have to make a sacrifice. Many older people adamantly refuse to move from their homes, even when it is no longer practical for them to live on their own. Most old folks fear entering a nursing home. Honestly, can you blame them? Some nursing homes should be feared. On the other hand, some caregivers have found great relief in being able to give up the caregiving role. Studies show that caregivers who place their charges in nursing homes improve their own health status. One caregiver describes the benefits of having her father in a nursing home as follows:

> The isolation that my dad experienced while living at home prevented the feeling of community for him. Creating community is one of the most important actions we can pursue for older adults, an action that supports people in the stage of their life when they need community to come to them, as it is sometimes difficult for them to "go to the community." It was easier for people to visit him when he lived in the care center, as they didn't have to fear finding him unconscious at home and they didn't have to worry about what they would do if he experienced the need for physical care during their visits.
>
> —Shirley Barnes, caregiver

Choosing the Least Unpleasant Option *Before* the Crisis Point

Making long-term care decisions is essentially a matter of picking the least unpleasant option. And most long-term care decisions are triggered by bad events. Caregivers rarely consider their options until the situation has reached a crisis point. Try to plan ahead. You do not want to have to make a decision in a crisis situation.

I am not suggesting that every person make a life plan for what to do if they need assistance. Such plans would probably be much too hypothetical and unrealistic. On the other hand, at a certain point in the long-term care journey you can see the horizon. You have to start asking how long the current voyage can be sustained. That is the time to start planning for what happens before the ship hits an iceberg. Making good decisions requires time, information, and clear goals. All sorts of emotions are aroused. Family conflicts may rekindle. You will make better decisions if you have an expert to support and guide you through the process.

Unfortunately, it is difficult to find unbiased assistance in making these difficult decisions. Most long-term care professionals have their own agendas. Hospital discharge planners' primary task is to move patients out of the hospital quickly. County caseworkers have to work under a budget, and have only a limited repertoire of services to promote. Still, before making a decision, try to talk it through with your care recipient, other family members, your doctors, and any other professionals you trust.

The Importance of Trust in Decision-Making

Trust can be a big issue in making long-term care decisions. Family members may be motivated by compassion and concern, or even guilt. Or they may seize the opportunity to get close to a weak older relative in order to access that relative's assets, or to influence bequests. In a situation where even family cannot automatically be trusted, letting a stranger into an older person's home to provide intimate care is even more challenging. Leaving a loved one in someone else's hands is a great act of trust. Do not feel uncomfortable about carefully monitoring the situation until a basis for that trust has been established.

Chapter One—Points to Ponder

Be prepared. Make sure this is really a role you can undertake. In some cases you may have no choice, but many times you do, even if it means pushing back on other family members or being prepared to spend money you would rather use for other things.

Be realistic. Caregiving takes endless patience and stamina. Pace yourself. You are in it for the long haul.

Protect yourself. Don't try to do it all. Ask for help. In fact, demand help from other family members. Find things they can do to share the burden.

Be organized. You will quickly become the center of a chaotic universe. You need to set up calendars to keep track of who is coming to do what tasks, doctor's appointments, and the like. You need careful records about medications and diagnoses. Every emergency room visit will be much easier (and ultimately safer) if you come prepared with a list of the older person's diagnoses, medications, and recent hospitalizations. Keep a careful list of each doctor, with contact information and when each visit occurred and what was done (see Chapter Three).

Do not assume. It is easy to believe that once you are in the hands of professionals they will do the right thing. But mistakes happen. Hospitals are dangerous places, and the best defense is vigilance. Doctors see many patients for short visits; lots can be overlooked during those brief encounters.

Ask questions. Medical professionals and long-term care personnel can be intimidating, but you cannot simply accept what they say. Be sure you understand all the instructions. Do not let yourself be hurried out the door without understanding what needs to be done. When changes in a care regimen are made, be sure you understand why. If something doesn't make sense, ask about it!

Choose your battles. You will see lots of things that are done less well than you would like, whether it is how a person cleans the house or prepares a meal, or whether nursing home staff seem as responsive as they should be. You need to stand up for older relatives, but you cannot constantly complain or your complaints will soon be dismissed.

Do not "overcare." Encourage the older person to do as much for herself as possible. It is easy to fall into the habit of doing things for her because it is faster and easier, but that behavior will encourage dependency. Older people need to be challenged, especially in small increments. You obviously do not want to push them too far, but try to push a little.

Respect the older person. Needing help from another person should not diminish the person in need. It is all too easy to infantilize frail older people. Try not to talk for them when you see the doctor. Listen to their opinions about decisions and take them seriously.

Be patient. This is much easier said than done, especially with persons with dementia who ask the same questions over and over. Try to find ways to change the subject or to divert them.

Reward yourself. You are undertaking invaluable work for your relative and your family. You may not always get acknowledgment from the older person or even from your own family. Give yourself a treat now and then.

Think ahead, plan, and be realistic. Making long-term care decisions and plans is hard but necessary.

Two

Money and the Law

One of the dirtiest words in the language of long-term care may be an unexpected one: money. The business of growing old is just that, a business, and a costly one. Medicare and Medigap[4] policies will cover many of the predictable costs—hospital bills and medical treatment—but other services like home care and personal care are generally not included. These personal-care services can make a big difference in the day-to-day life of frail older people, but many elders are reluctant to pay for such care. Older people have a penchant for putting off spending money, saving it for that proverbial "rainy day," but usually they want to save it to leave as a legacy.

Handling Conflicts over Paying for Care

Reluctance to pay for care can be the source of substantial family conflict. Even when their children beg them to use these services, some older individuals may refuse because they prefer to save their money for a real crisis or to be able to leave behind an inheritance. They may claim

---

4. Medigap is private insurance you can buy to cover some or all of the costs of medical care not covered by Medicare, largely the deductibles and copayments.

(even if they know better) that such services are unnecessary, or too costly, or that they should be covered by "the government" or private insurance. As a result, some elders will do whatever it takes to "get by" without paying for services and medical care. On the flip side, some adult children may prioritize preserving a legacy they view as their rightful, earned inheritance. This concern can lead children to guilt their aging parent about every penny spent, regardless of its necessity, or to make or influence decisions based on spending as little as possible.

In my own case, even though my sister and I had no interest in inheriting our mother's small estate, I found myself unwilling to spend money (her money) on her behalf in some situations. My sister pushed to buy more personal care, but I felt I was already paying for care from one source and resenting having to buy additional care. In retrospect, my sister was right; I probably had a false sense of justice. I should have put my mother's well-being first and not insisted the care system perform as it should.

Families resolve conflicts over paying for care in different ways. When all pleas are falling on parents' willfully deaf ears, sometimes the children will simply pay for the needed services themselves. Sometimes they will subsidize the costs of services and lead their parents to believe they cost less than they do. At other times the children will take on the burden of providing the care themselves until they become exhausted. The problem becomes especially tense when some children are willing to provide support but others will not or cannot. In the end, it is probably better to go ahead and pay for the needed care and then harangue your relatives to cover their share. You do not want to regret not having provided needed care. When conflicts cannot be resolved easily, a professional counselor or therapist may be helpful in mediating conversations between the adult siblings involved.

Medicare

The good news is that most older people are eligible for Medicare. The bad news is that Medicare does not pay for much long-term care. Medicare is basically a health insurance plan, and a very important one. The only reason a person would not be eligible for Medicare would be if he or she worked for federal or state governments some years ago or emigrated to this country and did not work enough years to qualify for Social Security. This means that for almost everyone, Medicare is an important part of paying for older people's health care. Almost everyone who is eligible for Social Security is eligible for Medicare. Although the age of eligibility for Social Security has been advanced slightly, Medicare eligibility begins at age sixty-five. For persons not still covered by private health insurance at age sixty-five there are penalties for delayed enrollment into the elective components (Parts B and D) of the program.

Medicare has three parts,* and making sense of what is and isn't covered can be challenging. Table 2.1 provides a quick summary.

Table 2.1: What Medicare Does and Does Not Pay For

Pays For	Does NOT Pay For
Hospital care	Long stays in nursing homes
Doctor visits	Assisted living
Lab tests	Home care
Rehabilitation, including short nursing home stays	Housing
Drugs (if you elect to enroll in Part D)	Personal assistance
Limited home health care	

Medicare Part A

Medicare Part A is essentially hospital insurance—including post-hospital care in rehabilitation units, nursing facilities, home health care,[5] and hospice care. Part A is automatically available to everyone sixty-five

---

5. As will become clear, home health care and home care are quite different, even though they look alike. Home health care is primarily a nursing service (delivered largely by aides) for medical conditions and their consequences, whereas home care is a social service that provides general assistance and support with a variety of activities.

* Part C refers to the provision to purchase managed care.

and older who is eligible for Social Security. Part A has some deductibles and copayments. The deductible is approximately equal to the cost of the first day of an acute care hospital stay. For very long hospital stays, there is a copayment. For nursing home stays that meet the Medicare requirements, the first twenty days are completely covered. After that, a sizable copayment is required. And if the stay exceeds one hundred days, the patient is completely responsible for the remaining costs. Many people have supplemental Medigap insurance plans (see page 50) that cover the deductible and other charges that Medicare approves but will not pay.

Medicare Part B

Part B of Medicare is medical insurance; it covers physician payments, therapies, laboratory test costs, and some associated costs. This coverage is optional, but because it is so heavily subsidized—the government pays about three-fourths of the bill—it is too good a deal to turn down. Part B can be purchased by anyone, even elders who are not eligible for Part A. The monthly premium for Part B is automatically deducted from Social Security payments.[6] There are deductibles and a 20 percent copayment.

Medicare Part D

The newest component of Medicare is Part D, which covers the cost of prescription drugs. Part D is an intimidating and complex program with a great deal of ambiguity. Many separate plans are available under this law. Although each plan is required to cover at least two drugs in defined categories, the actual drug types and brands covered will vary. Moreover, a plan may have multiple fee arrangements with varying patterns of coverage. Older people generally need a lot of help deciding which is the best provider of this drug insurance coverage. It is important to compare the drugs provided by a plan with those the elder is taking, and then shop for the best

6. People with low incomes who meet federal criteria are eligible for programs that pay some or all of their Medicare premiums and copayments.

price. There are computer programs to help in this selection, and many pharmacies will help. Like Part B, Part D is elective, but it is not as immediately clear if it is always a good deal. Part D's complicated payment formula has been nicknamed "the doughnut hole approach," and it works like this:

For drugs covered by your Part D plan, the patient pays:

- A monthly premium (varies depending on the plan you choose)[7]
- The first $275 per year for your prescriptions. This is called your deductible.

  After the $275 yearly deductible, here's how the costs work:
  - Patient pays 25 percent of yearly drug costs from $275 to $2,510, and the plan pays the other 75 percent of these costs, then
  - Patient pays 100 percent of your next $3,216.25 in drug costs,[8] then
  - Patient pays a coinsurance amount (about 5 percent of the drug cost) or a copayment (about $2.25 or $5.60 for each prescription) for the rest of the calendar year after the first $4,050 out-of-pocket (about $6,440 in total drug costs). The plan pays the rest.

The Patient Protection and Affordable Care Act of 2010 also provides for a 50 percent discount on brand-name drugs filled in the doughnut hole for persons with incomes less than $85,000 (couples $170,000).

When to Enroll in Part D

If you anticipate high drug costs for your parent, he or she obviously should enroll, but enrollment needs to happen when Medicare benefits begin. If your parent does not enroll in Part D at that time, there will be

---

7. The costs described here applied in 2010. They will likely change each year.
8. The Patient Protection and Affordable Care Act of 2010 provided a one-time extra payment of $250 to people who reach the coverage gap (doughnut hole). Beginning in 2011, the Act institutes a 50 percent discount on brand name drugs in the doughnut hole, and the Act will completely close the doughnut hole for all prescription drugs by 2020.

a penalty in the form of higher Medicare Part D premiums for each year enrollment has been delayed until they do decide to enroll.

Shopping for a Part D Carrier

Part D coverage comes from special drug benefit plans that are chartered by Medicare and are administered by private insurance companies or from enrollment in a Medicare managed care plan. Each drug benefit company may offer multiple plans with different copayments and deductibles, and each plan may cover different brands of drugs. Medicare requires that each plan offer at least two brands of each major drug type, but each plan's drug profile requires some scrutiny to make sure the drugs your parent is taking are covered by the plan of choice.

Match the Plan to the Drug Profile

Shopping for a Part D carrier can be exceptionally frustrating. The best approach is to look for the carrier that has a plan whose specific drug coverage most closely matches your parent's current drug profile. Computerized programs are available online from Medicare to help match a particular drug profile with those offered. The link to this site is provided in the appendix. You can also get help from most pharmacies, especially the big chains, who offer this service as an inducement to use their dispensing services.

Compare Cost

Chances are, your parent will need help[9] working with the programs and understanding all the variations involved. Many large pharmacy chains will also help customers select a Part D plan. After identifying plans that cover particular drugs, you must think about price. The basic premium is set by law, but because of the many variations in the programs offered, not all carriers charge the same fees. Some plans cover the

9. Chances are you will need help doing this, too.

minimal amounts set by law, but others help defray the costs of the out-of-pocket components as well. Obviously the greater the coverage, the more expensive the premium.

Annual Enrollment

Enrollment in Medicare Part D coverage requires subscribing to the same plan for one full year. It is possible to change coverage annually but not at other times. Even if your parent's medications change and the new prescriptions are not covered by your current Part D carrier, you cannot change plans except at the annual renewal period. Given that some prescriptions can cost hundreds of dollars each month, this can be a tremendous challenge for consumers.

Medigap

Because of the many deductibles and copayments lurking in the Medicare system, an insurance industry arose that sells what is called supplemental—or Medigap—insurance. A wide array of insurance programs cover some or all of the costs of deductibles and copayments. Some plans cover other services beyond the copayment coverage, such as preventive care or more posh accommodations. Some variations of Medigap plans previously offered drug programs, but many of these were eliminated when Part D was introduced. The range and description of each program is controlled by law. Each program must identify itself as fitting a predetermined type established by Medicare. As always, the greater the coverage, the steeper the price of the premium.

A serious pitfall of this system is purchasing multiple Medigap policies. Many older people are very concerned about having to pay out of pocket and often purchase several policies in the hopes of preventing this. This is a big mistake. In most cases, multiple policies simply cause duplicative coverage—they are a waste of money. The costs of the premiums for the separate plans can be higher than the dreaded deductibles. As with so many other money-based decisions, consumers need a reliable source of advice, someone who can sort out the options, explain the benefits and costs of each, and point out the perils of some choices. Family members can play that role if they have the time and patience to become knowledgeable, but given the complexity of the system, professional counselors are often a better solution.

Managed Care

When Medicare was enacted in 1965, it was designed to pay health care expenses on a fee-for-service basis. However, the modern-day health care system is a whole different animal. Many people are now covered by Medicare Advantage (Part C)—the Medicare program of managed care. These managed care programs can be big money-savers, but there are risks. Under these programs, the consumer pays a fixed monthly amount.[10] This covers all medical care needed during the month, as long as that care would be included in a typical Medicare program. Managed care programs also include a program based on Medicare Part D to cover prescription costs. Managed care can be a cheap alternative to purchasing supplemental insurance to cover costs not included in Medicare (deductibles and copayments; vision and hearing care; dentistry; podiatry, and so on). However, the amount of the monthly premium may be greater than the cost of premiums for Medicare Parts B and D, and the cost of copayments and deductibles for managed care vary. In parts of the country where Medicare costs are high, managed care companies may offer free services above and beyond Medicare requirements. Because the base price of Medicare Advantage reflects the average cost of fee-for-service care in an area, it is

---

10. The amount varies by location. In some settings, the underlying Medicare reimbursement is so high that the managed care programs offer additional services at no additional cost; all you pay is the Part B premium. In other places where the Medicare rates are much lower, additional care comes at an additional cost.

a good buy in areas where care is expensive. Conversely, in areas where care is cheaper, a substantial additional payment is usually required.

The costs of Medicare Advantage plans are likely to increase in response to payment revisions mandated by the Patient Protection and Affordable Care Act of 2010, which reduced the subsidies to such plans, bringing them into line with the costs of fee-for-service care.

Restricted Choice in Managed Care

As parents grow older, their needs and care providers will shift in unpredictable ways. Managed care provides them with a clearly organized care system that can make it simpler to choose a doctor or a course of treatment. But this is not necessarily a good thing. Managed care simplifies decisions by offering a smaller set of options. The choice of health care providers may be limited, or the plan may require special permission to visit out-of-network doctors. Not everyone welcomes such restrictions. Most managed care plans restrict the options for care, and even if it is possible to visit a doctor or specialist outside the network, patients may be required to cough up large copayments for that privilege. Before your parent enrolls in a managed care program, take the time to make sure that she will be able to continue to visit any trusted doctors.

"Cherry Picking" in Managed Care

As with much of the health care system, managed care companies are primarily in the business of making a profit. Because you pay a fixed amount for care each month, managed care companies are constantly tempted to treat only those who are healthiest. This practice is sometimes called "cherry picking." Some managed care companies offer rewards, like gym memberships, to attract healthier clients. Another concern is that managed care companies will seek to maximize their profits by denying necessary care or by using cheap and ineffective care. However, supporters of managed care claim that because good care can prevent expensive treatment for serious problems, it is ultimately cheaper. The jury is still out on whether managed care is a good buy. It may be for some people and not others. If you are considering it, be sure to understand just what you are getting and what you will be expected to pay for that care.

Switching from Managed Care to a Supplemental Plan May Pose Challenges

One last thing to bear in mind when weighing the pros and cons of managed care is that although you can easily un-enroll from Medicare managed care, it may be hard to repurchase supplemental insurance. The prices of coverage may have soared, or you may be disqualified altogether because of a new or intensified illness. Resources with additional information on Medicare Advantage plans are available in the appendix.

Medicaid

Another government-run program that pays some of the costs of long-term care is Medicaid. Unlike Medicare, which is open to everyone over the age of sixty-five, Medicaid is designed to cover the medical costs of low-income families and older persons. Medicaid covers some things not included in the Medicare program, like long-term care and some medical care (hearing aids, for example).

Qualifying for Medicaid

There are two ways to qualify for Medicaid. First, anyone who is already included in the welfare system (because of poverty or severe disability) is entitled to Medicaid. Second, depending on what state you live in, a person whose medical costs spike beyond a preset percentage of total income may be declared Medically Needy. That means Medicaid assistance will cover all health care costs above that preset percentage of income. The definitions of Medically Needy vary from state to state; not every state has this category of eligibility program. The most direct way to find out about the eligibility rules in your state is to call the local welfare office. Alternatively, you can consult a lawyer or financial planner who specializes in aging, or you may be able to get help from the social work department in your local hospital.

Basically, your parent is expected to shell out her own money first; then Medicaid will step in and pick up the rest of the bill. The benchmarks of medical need change from state to state. In order to be declared Medically Needy, one's income and assets must be below certain levels. Homes and cars are not usually included as assets, assuming we are not talking about a collection of cars or a string of vacation homes. However, the income and asset levels are set differently in different states. Medicaid is a mixed federal and state program. The federal government matches state dollars at levels from about 50 percent for the richer states to 95 percent for the poorer ones. The federal government sets minimum standards for eligibility and benefits for each state's Medically Needy program. But with federal permission, the states can go beyond those levels to make them more inclusive. Some states have programs to cover the "near poor"—the large number of people who are just above the federal poverty level. In other states, however, no Medically Needy program has been put in place. The Patient Protection and Affordable Care Act of 2010 broadens income eligibility for Medicaid and may make it easier for some older people to qualify.

Doing the Medicaid Math

Once you learn the rules that pertain in your state, you can do some quick math to see if your family member qualifies as Medically Needy. Identify how much of her income she is allowed to keep after paying for room and board and medical care. Add up her current expenses and subtract from her income. She may be required to sell her assets and convert them to income. If expenses exceed a predetermined portion of income, the rest is covered by Medicaid. However, "the rest" must now meet Medicaid definitions of eligible services. If a person is covered by Medicaid because she qualifies for welfare, Medicaid coverage will not change unless she becomes ineligible for welfare. But if a person is covered for Medicaid because she is Medically Needy, she must be recertified each month. The concept of Medically Needy is heavily biased toward nursing home care because it is easier to predict nursing homes' monthly costs and so families know in advance if they qualify for Medicaid. Because home care costs are more likely to go up and down from month to month, older people do not automatically qualify each month and the entitlement process is more complicated. This has unfortunately led many families to place Medically Needy Medicaid recipients in nursing homes.

Medicaid and Nursing Homes, Home Health, and Other Care

Nursing home care and home health care are mandatory parts of all state Medicaid programs. Other forms of community care, however, such as personal-care attendants and assisted living, are not always available. States have the option of applying to the federal government for special community care waivers. These allow them to use money that would have been spent on nursing home care to provide community-based services. These waivers may also allow the state to offer community care services in some regions of the state and not others, depending on the priorities and preferences of regional Agencies on Aging. Things may be getting better for community-based long-term care (LTC). The Patient Protection and Affordable Care Act of 2010 broadens states' ability to use Medicaid funds for community care.

The waiver programs vary from state to state. Each program has specific eligibility rules and may have waiting lists. It is usually necessary to get some form of professional assistance to seek care under waivers. Local federally funded Area Agencies on Aging are a good place to start. They are found in almost every county (and there is a national 800 number: 800-677-1116). Financial eligibility for waiver programs is more generous than the basic Medicaid services, often two to three times the basic Medicaid threshold.

Medicaid eligibility and services range from stingy to generous from state to state. Medicaid is never allowed to pay more for nursing home care than private rates. In two states, Minnesota and North Dakota, the rates are identical for private pay and Medicaid, but in most states Medicaid pays considerably less. This means that nursing home residents who pay for their care with private means can get better accommodations and more services than Medicaid recipients. But even for private pay residents, nursing home life is neither gracious nor overstaffed.

Families can boost the quality of care for persons on Medicaid by purchasing services over and above what Medicaid covers. Again, the rules permitting this additional care vary by state. In many states it is possible to hire private duty attendants or to pay for a private room, but some states view these special services as equivalent to income. So adding these services may cause an older person who previously qualified as Medically Needy to become ineligible.

Spousal Protection

Spousal protection allows older couples greater financial freedom to deal with the challenges of Alzheimer's in the most comfortable way possible. If an older person with Alzheimer's disease begins to rack up high medical costs, they can be determined Medically Needy even if their husband's or wife's finances are outside the typical limit. Basically, Medicaid overlooks the ownership of a house and a certain amount of income and assets. This allows one spouse to continue to live at home, even if Medicaid is financing a nursing home stay for the spouse with Alzheimer's. The Patient Protection and Affordable Care Act of 2010 mandates that states include spousal impoverishment protections in Medicaid waiver programs.

Dual Eligibles

Some people who are Medicare beneficiaries are also eligible for Medicaid. These "dual eligibles" have very complete coverage. Not only does Medicaid pay for Medicare's deductibles and copayments, it also covers services that are outside of the Medicare system. As you might have guessed, those who are eligible for both systems typically need more medical care and have greater expenses than those who are not.

Divestiture

Although Medicaid was created to supplement the welfare program, many older people and their families have come to see it as a right. After paying taxes for years to support it, they feel they deserve some rewards. Because one route to Medicaid eligibility is becoming Medically Needy, some older adults with modest incomes and sufficient assets to protect may be tempted to divest themselves of assets to become eligible. Divestiture—which means parents turning over all assets to their children—has become a common occurrence.

No one really knows just how prevalent this practice actually is, but many lawyers and financial planners now specialize in this form of estate planning. Even if an older person or their family is reluctant to take advantage of the system unless their situation is desperate, estate planners may encourage families to manipulate their finances in order to qualify for Medicaid.

Medicaid has responded to this threat by creating the "look back" system. The rules vary among states, but the gist of it is that after the beneficiary dies, Medicaid can claim some of the costs of care from the heirs. The underlying rationale is that Medicaid is entitled to any money given to family members or non-charitable organizations in the three to five years just before the beneficiary was declared Medically Needy. The "look back" procedure for recovering Medicaid costs varies from state to state, and as divestiture grows more popular, Medicaid looks further and further back into beneficiaries' financial histories.

Divestiture not only opens up the possibility that Medicaid will claim part of a person's estate after death, it also leaves an older person vulnerable. When parents turn over all assets to their children, they are then entirely dependent on the assumption that their children will continue to look after them. And timing can be tricky. When a parent divests money near the time of his death, his family may be taxed heavily. Such a step means giving over great control to the recipients. It is an act of profound trust that should be honored.

Unplanned events can complicate things. For example, if the assets are turned over to a son or daughter for management on the elder person's behalf, they become part of common property in the case of an acrimonious divorce.

Hiring Financial and Legal Counsel for Divestiture

There are professionals who specialize in helping older people avoid taxes and become eligible for Medicaid. The latter is easier in some states than others. Most states have tightened their eligibility rules as money has gotten tighter, and the "look back" procedure continues to reach further into a person's financial history. States may also attach liens (or at least claims) to property like homes, to be applied when the older person has died. These can make probate more complicated. If someone is to be hired to provide financial and legal counsel for your parent to become Medicaid eligible, be sure the professional is truly competent. In this case, word of mouth is probably all you can go by, but you may be interested in their philosophy as well.

Ethics of Divestiture

This issue of becoming Medicaid eligible raises a number of personal, logistical, and even moral questions. Some people view manipulating one's assets and income to appear in greater need as deceptive and frankly wrong. Others have a strong sense of entitlement to Medicaid support, arguing they have paid taxes for many years and now it is their turn to dip into the trough.

I prefer to duck the moral and ethical innuendos and focus on the pragmatic. If your parent does plan to divest, you need to do two things.

Number one, start early. Not only does the state look back up to five years when assessing eligibility, precipitous divestment raises all sorts of red flags. Number two, be sure you absolutely trust whomever your parent is handing over assets to; they will own these assets and your parent's options. This sort of divestiture is a big step financially and emotionally. It puts the older person in a position of dependency from which they cannot emerge. It threatens their autonomy and self-image.

Private Long-Term Care Insurance

Those who can afford to may want to purchase private long-term care (LTC) insurance. This allows a person to avoid the complicated Medicare and Medicaid systems while protecting private assets. Until recently, the only option to purchase long-term care insurance was through a private company. Some employers have arranged some form of group purchase (without necessarily subsidizing the cost), which may yield some discount on the premium; the employees pay the full cost if they elect to purchase such coverage.

Recent legislation may change the landscape of private LTC insurance. The Patient Protection and Affordable Care Act of 2010 includes a provision called CLASS (Community Living Assistance Services and Supports), which provides a national voluntary LTC insurance program that pays a cash benefit to individuals who are unable to perform ADLs; this benefit can be used to purchase community-based services. Details are still being developed; the benefit is modest (about $50 a day), but it could form the basis for LTC planning. It should encourage the development of more community-based services.

The decision about buying long-term care insurance is complicated. Like all insurance it is a combination of saving and investment. The arguments in favor are essentially protecting assets (leaving a larger legacy) and being able to afford better care. A person has guaranteed eligibility at the time of enrollment. Delaying until a condition emerges may mean that they are no longer eligible. The arguments against are the cost. It involves expending disposable income on a product that will not be needed for some time. This money might be better invested to yield a higher return. For some people, the goal is to preserve their assets, presumably to leave as a legacy. For others, the tipping point is the aversion to going on Medicaid, which they see as a stigmatized welfare program.

If Buying Private Insurance, Buy Early (But Not Too Early)

The industry is still evolving, but it works about the same way as any other form of insurance. Consumers can decide at any age to buy the insurance. The younger the consumer, the lower the premium (but the lower the likelihood of any use in the foreseeable future). The earlier you buy such care, the longer you will wait to use it and the greater the chance that new forms of care will arise that may not be specifically addressed in the benefits package.

The insurance companies do not take big risks. They carefully screen applicants to eliminate those most likely to need long-term care. If your family member plans on purchasing private insurance, it is best to buy early (but not too early); most plans are purchased by people in their late sixties. Aside from the fact that premium costs climb with age, waiting too long may lead to lack of eligibility. Certain diseases could be roadblocks for long-term care insurance or could drive the premium costs too high.

Working the Private Insurance System

Sometimes consumers can dodge insurance company restrictions by applying to be part of a group plan. However, this option is usually only made available to employee groups, so most frail older persons are not able to cheat the system and use group plans to purchase affordable private insurance. Since most people will not need long-term care until they are well into their eighties, buying private insurance is really just a system of saving up for that care. Long-term care insurance is essentially term insurance. Once the premiums have been paid, there is no way of recovering the money. Another option with more flexibility is to set aside money in investments. The investments can provide for care down the road, but are also recoverable in the event that the care is not needed, or not needed to the extent of investment value.

Pros and Cons of Long-Term Care Plans

Long-term care insurance policies offer a varying range of benefits. The most important difference is that some policies cover the costs of a set of care options, while others provide money for treatment costs directly to the insured. Plans that pay cash send a case manager to assess the condition and confirm the need for treatment. Service-based plans skip this step but charge a sizable copayment or deductible. For example, a service-based insurance company might pay the costs of a nursing home stay—but the patient has to pay the first 25 percent. If your parent is considering a service-based policy, make sure it covers as many care options (especially the choice of home care or assisted-living care) as possible. It's better to purchase a plan that makes cash payments if you can. Service coverage policies may restrict the covered services to only those provided by a certified agency. Care from such an agency may be much more expensive that what you could buy directly from a personal attendant you hired, rendering the financial protection from the insurance moot.

How can a person know at age fifty what types of services will be important to have covered thirty-five years later or even what the long-term care services of the future will look like? This uncertainty is the biggest conundrum people face when considering buying long-term care coverage. The world of long-term care is changing too quickly to make worthwhile predictions. Even if someone purchases a cash-based policy, buying private insurance is an uncertain investment. Say a person is in her fifties and considering purchasing private long-term care insurance. She's not likely to see payments from this policy until her mid-eighties. Rising inflation rates guarantee that thirty-five years from now, what was a generous payment will be small pennies. So cash-based policies have to find a way to adjust for inflation. Unfortunately, this raises the costs considerably.

Even if you are willing to take a chance on evolving types of care and climbing inflation rates, there is another important factor in the private insurance equation—the role of government funding. The costs you insure today may be covered by the government in the future (either through Medicaid or universal LTC insurance such as that promised in the 2010 Patient Protection and Affordable Care Act). On the flip side, government funding may dwindle away, meaning that good private insurance plans will become crucial, and more expensive.

Some states have a special program called Partnership, whereby if you buy long-term care insurance the state will waive an amount equivalent to your coverage in calculating your allowable assets for determining your Medicaid eligibility under the Medically Needy category described above.

More resources discussing the pros and cons of private long-term care insurance are available in the appendix.

Using Life Insurance to Buy Care

There are several ways a person can use life insurance as an asset to pay for long-term care and associated costs. Your parent can, in essence, sell her life insurance benefits to a third party. She will get the discounted value of the face value of the policy. The purchaser becomes liable for all future premium payments. She is thereby reducing her estate by converting some of its latent value into cash.

Viatical Settlements

A variation of the life settlement is the viatical settlement. Whereas the life settlement is usually negotiated when a person is reasonably healthy and has some life expectancy, the viatical settlement is designed for end-of-life care. The insured person must have a life expectancy of two years or less. The benefits are sold to a viatical company that pays a discounted rate. Do not enter into either of these negotiations lightly, and discuss them with a knowledgeable financial advisor.

Accelerated Death Benefits

Some life insurance policies offer an accelerated death benefit option, which pays a cash advance on the death benefit while the insured person is still alive. It is essentially a loan against the cash value of the policy.

Homes as Collateral (Reverse Mortgages)

A person's home is her castle. It is also often her largest asset. Financial planners (both scrupulous and not) have recognized this fact and have proposed ways to convert this asset into cash that can be used to support older people through their final years. This money might be used to pay for home care, for example. The average eighty-year-old is not a good candidate for a traditional mortgage because he or she has no way of paying back the loan. The basic idea of a reverse mortgage is essentially to sell the house in advance but to allow the seller to then live in it rent free until they die or need institutional care. The price represents a discount that is presumably based on the costs of the new buyer postponing taking possession right away. The elderly seller receives a lump sum payment that they can use however they want. Many purchase arrangements also induce the seller to put the money in some type of annuity, which guarantees them a fixed income. But there is no reason to couple the annuity purchase with the house sale and you may be able to find better deals elsewhere.

The Drawbacks of Reverse Mortgages

Although reverse mortgages might seem like a good idea, most studies suggest they are not. The net value taken out of the house may be substantially less than the market value. There are lots of costs and charges frequently associated with the transaction. The associated annuities may prove poor investments. Here again, your parent needs competent professional assistance from someone who is clearly an advocate for your parent.

Sometimes the reverse mortgage works to the older person's advantage. The longest lived person on record is a Frenchwoman who sold her house under a variation of a reverse mortgage and outlived the person who bought it.

Estate Planning

Older people must put their houses in order, but there are lots of reasons to put it off. I personally found it extremely frightening to sit down and make explicit plans about how my own estate (a rather lofty term) should be handled upon my death. It meant actually admitting out loud that I was going to die, a fact I repress with great fervor. One of my favorite Woody Allen quotes is, "I don't want to achieve immortality through my work. I want to achieve it through not dying." Ultimately a strong sense of responsibility (and a persistent wife) caused me to acknowledge the need to take active steps. Once my wife and I met with an attorney (preferably find one who does this sort of work as a major part of her job), I came to realize how important it is to have a clear will and the associated planning that goes with it. The alternative is to die without a will and leave your relatives to enter probate.

Probate is the process of legally deciding who should receive what. It is much more expeditiously accomplished if the deceased person has left instructions, particularly legally binding ones. Things have likely improved since Dickensian times, but anyone putting off estate planning should be obliged to read *Bleak House*. Table 2.2 summarizes available options for funding care.

Good Help Is Essential in Estate Planning

Estate planning means both taking stock of what you have and deciding how you want to distribute it. It may also involve making plans for your

Table 2.2: Coverage Comparison of Available Financing Options

FINANCE OPTION	CHARACTERISTIC					
	Only Available for Long– Term Costs	Remaining Funds Available to Heirs	Rate of Asset Accumulation	Eligibility Requirement	Risk of Insufficient Funds	Cost
Family Support— Caregiving	No	No	None	No	Moderate family support— caregiving	You pay for services— family member
Personal Savings	Yes	Yes	Variable	No	High long-term care costs can exceed your personal savings	You are respon- sible for creating private savings
Long-Term Care Insurance	Yes	No	Fixed	Yes	Moderate to low long-term care costs could exceed original cover- age amount	Monthly premiums for the life of the policy
Limited Long-Term Care Insurance	Yes	No	Fixed	Yes	Moderate to low amount received from benefit may not pay all long-term care costs	None
Life Settlement	Yes	No	Fixed	Yes	Moderate to low amount received from benefit may not pay all long-term care costs	None
Viatical Settlement	Yes	No	Fixed	Yes	Moderate to low amount received from benefit may not pay all long-term care cost	None

Table 2.2 (continued)

FINANCE OPTION	CHARACTERISTIC					
	Only Available for Long-Term Costs	Remaining Funds Available to Heirs	Rate of Asset Accumulation	Eligibility Requirement	Risk of Insufficient Funds	Cost
Accelerated Death Benefit	Yes	No	Fixed	Yes	Moderate to low amount received from benefit may not pay all long-term care costs	None
Reverse Mortgages	No	Yes	Variable	Yes	Moderate amount received from benefit may not pay all long-term care costs. Home maintenance costs still exist	Processing and origination fee to establish mortgage
Continuing Care Retirement Community	Yes	Yes	Variable	Yes	Low additional care provided as needed in CCRC assisted-living or nursing facility	High purchase price and fixed monthly payment
Veterans Benefits	No	No	None	Yes	Moderate to high amount received from benefit may not pay all long-term care costs	None

Table 2.2 (continued)

FINANCE OPTION	CHARACTERISTIC					
	Only Available for Long–Term Costs	Remaining Funds Available to Heirs	Rate of Asset Accumulation	Eligibility Requirement	Risk of Insufficient Funds	Cost
Medicare	No	No	None	Yes	Moderate to high amount received from Medicare may not pay all long-term care costs	Copayments and deductibles. You are responsible for creating private savings
Medicaid	No	No	None	Yes	High amount received from Medicaid may not pay all long-term care costs; recovery of Medicaid may be made against estate	You pay for services not covered by Medicaid
PACE	Yes	No	None	Yes	Moderate to high amount received from benefit may not pay all long-term care costs	You pay for services not covered by PACE

Source: Janet Gibson, *The Complete Guide for Senior Care* (Minneapolis: WiseLife Press, 2007).

own financial security. Because the inheritance tax laws keep changing, your parent should discuss this topic with someone skilled and up-to-date. There may be many options; many have tax consequences. Some involve making bequests well before death to avoid inheritance tax (which may vary widely depending upon the year of death, it seems). Early bequests may come when adult children can use them, but they obviously should not be made if your parent cannot afford them. A panoply of devices is available, including trusts. This is not a do-it-yourself project. Good help is essential. Be prepared that such help will be expensive.

Anticipate Questions in Dividing the Estate

When it comes to deciding how an estate should be divided, all sorts of issues emerge. What principle of fairness will be employed? Should each child receive according to need? Should the division be equal? How do grandchildren figure into the calculation? What happens if some of your children are more prolific than others? Are some people more deserving because of what they did? There are no easy or correct answers. Each strategy has consequences. But so does doing nothing. Some parents do well with discussing questions and issues directly with their adult children, and this may be something you can encourage your parent to do.

Some older people obsess over their wills, making (or at least planning) changes on a regular basis. It may become a pastime.

Advance Directives

The hottest topic in the long-term care world in recent years has been end-of-life care. This touchy topic generates many ethical questions, especially surrounding "futile" care—care that has little or no chance of improving a person's health status. Advance directives are becoming more and more common. Advance directives are written statements that give people a way to voice opinions about treatments they would or wouldn't want, even if they aren't able to communicate their wishes at the time. So, even if a person were in a coma, or had advanced dementia or some form of aphasia (the inability to speak or express ideas) after a stroke, he can still have control over what happens to him.

I have some personal philosophical issues with advance directives on several levels. First, it seems bitterly ironic that we appear to give more autonomy to the comatose than the conscious. Why should we expect that the desires of people in a coma will be followed when the care system often ignores the preferences of those who are alert? Second, the values we hold about states of disability are often flawed. Most people overly fear life with severe disability. Our society is crammed with exaggerated beliefs about how much (or how little) disability and illness a person can willingly tolerate. A person who is healthy and independent might think life would be miserable in a dependent or immobile condition.

But in reality, most people deal with increasing frailty without much difficulty and find meaning in lives they may have thought would be unbearable when they were well. It is almost impossible for a person to imagine how she would feel about so-called futile care until the choice is upon her. We are more adaptable than we think we are. Studies that have compared the values placed on life with disability by those with and without the disability show consistently that those who are currently free of disability place a much more negative weight on being disabled. As Shakespeare's Macbeth says, "Present fears are less than horrible imaginings." This means that we may too heavily discount the value of care in some imagined state and argue against care in the abstract.

For this reason, I distinguish advance directives from end-of-life decisions. Advance directives are based on beliefs about how a patient will feel and what she would want under certain hypothetical circumstances. By contrast, end-of-life decisions refer to decisions made by persons who are already experiencing the situation, not imagining what it would be like. They are in a good position to weigh the alternatives and decide if they want to continue in this state. Their decisions are based on actual experience. An older person who is in intractable pain or is paralyzed knows just what it feels like to be that way. They are better positioned to decide how much of such a state they are prepared to bear. All too often the rest of us are less prepared for that decision. We have tools at hand to counter these expressed preferences. It might be helpful to check out the movie *Whose Life Is It Anyway?* which describes the efforts of a young artist who is paralyzed to forgo further treatment. The clinical staff label him as depressed and take him to court. We talk a lot about respecting older people's preferences, but it can be very painful to have to live up to those principles.

Nonetheless, advance directives are being heavily promulgated, and it is useful to understand them.

Forms of Advance Directives

Advance directives can take several forms. The two most common choices are to make a living will, or to appoint a durable medical power of attorney. There are pros and cons to each option. Even for those who would rather leave it to fate, it never hurts to consider the question. Federal law requires hospitals and nursing homes to give all incoming patients the opportunity to voice their end-of-life preferences. The forms can come as a grim surprise. They usually present a list of treatments, almost like a menu. The patient can order up the course of treatment they find most palatable. Although all patients must be offered such menus, completing the forms is optional. Some states (including Vermont and Rhode Island) have developed more humane approaches. Many hospitals and nursing homes use the widely available Five Wishes form. It essentially asks for five things:

1. The Person I Want to Make Care Decisions for Me When I Can't
2. My Wish for the Kind of Medical Treatment I Want or Don't Want
3. My Wish for How Comfortable I Want to Be

4. My Wish for How I Want People to Treat Me

5. My Wish for What I Want My Loved Ones to Know

Resources providing more information on the Five Wishes form are listed in the appendix.

The Five Wishes form is immediately accepted as a legal document in most states. This is important. Typically, state-specific documents are not legally binding outside the state in which they were completed. Whatever approach you choose to take, it is best to have a plan in place before you enter a hospital or nursing home.

POLST: Physician Orders for Life-Sustaining Treatment

Another stage in advance directives is the Physician Orders for Life-Sustaining Treatment (POLST), a program being organized by physicians in several states. POLST is basically a set of standing orders completed by a physician after consultation with the patient and her family. The intent behind POLST is to make end-of-life orders the norm instead of the exception. The purpose is to document preferences about end-of-life care explicitly, translate those wishes into physician's orders, and thereby allow staff to act in the absence of a physician. POLST documents can be used to specifically order the limitation of treatment, to order no treatment, or to order full treatment. The orders specify the type and amounts of treatment to be given under various circumstances, including hospitalization, resuscitation, tube feeding, intravenous fluids, and antibiotics. And the orders are supposed to follow the patient wherever she goes. At least in theory, EMTs seeing such orders prominently displayed would refrain from starting unwanted CPR if they had a doctor's orders to refer to.

Discuss Preferences Sooner Rather Than Later

Sometimes older people are reluctant to discuss these preferences. But more often, families are reluctant to broach the topic, even when older people are quite comfortable talking about death. Some older people derive great solace from discussing their death and especially their legacy. They may make endless lists of what should be given to whom. Some even design their funeral arrangements in great detail. Some use this as an opportunity to work through many of the events and relationships in their lives and bring some closure (even if it may mean reinventing history). Aging usually brings people a greater comfort with their own mortality. It is better to have conversations about end-of-life preferences before it is too late. A serious problem can arise when older persons enter an advanced stage of dementia before they have made their preferences known. It is important to have these discussions while your loved one is still able to clearly and rationally express herself.

Ensure That Directives Are Carried Out

Ironically, despite all the attention lavished on getting people to create advance directives, and federal laws mandating that everyone be given the chance to state their end-of-life preferences, these preferences are routinely ignored. Medical care centers are always anxious to avoid litigation. Health care providers are reluctant to forgo treatment if they sense any conflict within the family. They do not want to open themselves up to the possibility of a lawsuit from a disgruntled family member. So whether your parent has expressed a wish for "heroic measures" or "letting go," in order for those advance directives to be carried out, you must make sure the whole family is aware of the preferences and agrees to go along with those wishes. Even if a parent has signed over durable power of attorney for health to an adult child and is considered incapable of truly informed consent, doctors and nurses are still likely to seek "assent" from a person with dementia for surgical procedures and the like. Although technically they should not have to bother, a bit of reflection would suggest that a cooperative rather than a protesting patient is important. Subjecting someone to anesthesia or invasive procedures feels like assault to those on both sides of the transaction.

Patients Can Change Their Minds About Advance Directives

It is important to remember that advance directives have no legal force if the patient is conscious and aware and able to state a preference. No one is obliged to follow his or her own advance directives, thank goodness! The even greater irony is that some health professionals seem to pay more attention to what people who can no longer express an opinion said in advance than to the expressed opinions of those still quite conscious. It may prove very difficult to get some clinicians to truly hear what a patient wants, especially if they do not agree with that course.

Living Wills

A living will is one of the most popular ways to create advance directives. Basically, a living will lists the actions you wish to have happen or do not wish to have happen (resuscitation, admission to the hospital, use of antibiotics, and so on) should you ever be unable to voice your end-of-life preferences. Despite the current push for living wills, you should carefully consider what it means for your parent to make a will stating a wish not to receive intense care. Basically, your parent is giving up opportunities for care. Is your parent sure she wants to commit to a limited menu of possible treatments? A person might regret the choice to forgo care. Sometimes, the best option is a more general written statement from a person about what matters most in life, and a description of the way he would like to live.

If your parent chooses to make a living will, it is worthless unless steps are taken to make sure it will be available when needed. What are the chances that the emergency medical technicians (EMTs) called to handle an emergency will take the time to look for a living will? One solution is something called the Vial of Life Project. The "vials" provide EMTs with information about allergies, medication regimens, and end-of-life preferences. The Vial of Life Project's website address is provided in the appendix.

Durable Power of Attorney

Appointing someone with durable health care power of attorney is a better and more flexible way to deal with advance directives. Durable powers of attorney can cover many issues. The most crucial distinction is between a power of attorney form that assigns control over financial matters and a form designating someone to act as an older person's agent if she loses the power to act for herself in making health care decisions. A person can do either without the other or both, if desired. If an older person chooses to draw up a durable power of attorney for health care (DPOAH) form, careful attention should be given to the decision of which person will speak for the patient if she is unable to do so. The designated person—whether you or someone else—should be someone who knows your relative well, including his values and general medical and end-of-life preferences. The person should be a trusted individual, and, ideally, one who does not stand to benefit directly from the patient's death.

It's important for everyone involved to be part of the discussions, but health care providers cannot tolerate multiple "agents," so someone must be selected. Not everything can be anticipated in advance, however; the main advantage of a DPOAH over a living will is that it allows a proxy decision-maker to take into account the actual particulars of the health emergency and the medical information. If there are several possible candidates for DPOAH, it is best if the agent lives near the older person so as to be closer in an emergency. Also, some families prefer to designate the DPOAH to a person with medical or nursing background, if there is such a person. Although a spouse should always be involved, some elderly persons would prefer one of their children be the agent for both parents and may become jittery with advance directive discussions.

It's also important to know that such discussions are not binding. A patient's preferences in real time trump any statements she may have made earlier. The person appointed as the durable power of attorney for health cannot overrule the patient when she is awake and aware. Remember, a patient is never required to follow his or her own advance directives. It is everyone's prerogative to change his or her mind.

Patients Can Speak for Themselves

There is something painfully ironic about all this attention to advance directives. It is as if we placed more value on the lives of comatose people than those who are alert. Why are we not showering the same level of attention on helping people make informed decisions every day about care in real time?

It is important to understand the difference between end-of-life decisions and advance directives. Advance directives are statements of preferences about what treatment a patient would and would not want under various circumstances. Advance directives take effect only when the patient is unable to competently express end-of-life wishes. If the patient can express a preference, it does not matter what he wrote out in advance directives. He may have made prior statements about not wanting any extraordinary treatment, but if he is able to speak for himself when the time comes, he is free to change his mind.

Chapter Two—Points to Ponder

Money is important. You can buy more and better care with more money.

Do not skimp. In the long run you will be happier knowing you did what you could to make the older person as comfortable as possible.

Money has to last. At the same time, it is hard to estimate how long the need for long-term care may go on. Realistic budgeting is needed.

Public programs are available. Take advantage of what is out there.

Get help. You will need professional guidance to understand what an older person is entitled to.

Consider long-term care insurance. Weigh the options. Decide how risk averse you are and what your and your parent's financial goals are.

Plan for the end of life. Don't be afraid to discuss the topic. Older people are likely to be more comfortable with the conversation than you.

Listen to your loved one. Talk to the older person about what they want. Encourage discussions about how much care they will want in moments of crisis. At least get a sense of their perception of their sense of their quality of life.

Consider a durable power of attorney for health. It is important to have access to your parent's financial accounts and to be designated as a decision-maker if a crisis should arise and she became unable to communicate her wishes.

Three

Finding a Good Doctor

As the name implies, long-term care is an ongoing process. Most people receiving long-term care have serious medical conditions. This means medical personnel will play a major role in their remaining years. So choosing a doctor is very important. But finding the right doctor can be very hard. Most doctors don't specialize in diagnosing and treating older patients. This makes finding a good doctor for an older person much harder and yet all the more necessary. Ideally, you should find a geriatrician, a physician who is specially trained in the care of older persons.

Finding a Geriatrician

Geriatricians are physicians who have received special additional training in how to diagnose and manage diseases of older people. They are very rare and becoming rarer despite the demographic revolution in which the eighty-five-and-over set is the fastest growing cohort in the American population. Geriatricians do not practice to get rich. On average, they earn about $150,000 a year, which is less than half the roughly $400,000 of a doctor practicing a specialty such as radiology. The relatively low level of payment may be one reason why few physicians have been attracted to geriatrics as a career. Another is because it is hard work. Dealing with frail older patients can be demanding and not everyone is cut out for such a practice.

The typical symptoms of many medical conditions change dramatically with age. For example, complaints of chest pain are a classic sign of a heart attack, but an older person suffering a heart attack may instead become confused and agitated. Doctors trained in classic cases may misinterpret these symptoms. So whenever possible, an older patient should be evaluated by a geriatrician.

To find the names of geriatricians in your area, you can contact the American Geriatrics Society (contact information for the AGS is included in the appendix). The AGS will give you the names of accredited geriatricians.

Check with Your Local Hospital

Besides contacting the American Geriatrics Society, another option for helping your parent locate a geriatrician is to call local hospitals to see if they have a geriatrics department. Be sure to ask about the credentials of the geriatricians on staff. Geriatricians have undergone special additional training and have passed special examinations. Especially outside of urban areas, a geriatrics department may not be staffed by specially trained and board-certified geriatricians. If your parent lives near a medical school, you can call there to find out whether they have a geriatrics training program. These programs are designed to give physicians special geriatrics training beyond their usual training and residency. If the school has a geriatrics training program, the physicians training there (and the faculty supervising them) often staff the clinics. Check to see if the clinic is "referral only." This means a primary care clinician must refer your parent to the geriatrician; patients cannot "self-refer." Many geriatrics programs allow patients (or more typically families) to self-refer because other physicians are reluctant to do so.

When You Can't Locate a Geriatrician: Primary Care Physicians

The highest hurdle between your parent and good geriatric care is the shortage of geriatricians. Even if there is a geriatrician in the area, there may be no openings for new patients in their practice. Another option is to find a good primary care doctor, especially one who specializes in caring for older people, or at least likes to care for such patients. But finding a good primary care doctor can be almost as challenging as finding a geriatrician. The local medical society can provide names, but they cannot offer information on who specializes in older people or how good they are. Your parent's friends can be a better resource; they can recommend doctors they like but may not be in a good position to judge the doctors' competence.

If you are able to help your parent find a good primary care doctor, he or she may not accept new patients, especially patients on Medicare. Medicare does not pay well for ambulatory care, so doctors can be reluctant to take on Medicare patients, or they may have opted out of Medicare altogether. Aside from the issue of Medicare, evaluating an older patient takes a lot of time. Many older patients have several problems and may communicate slowly. Doctors get paid by the visit, regardless of how long the visit lasts. One response could be to schedule multiple visits and treat one problem at a time, but this strategy conflicts with one of the main goals of geriatrics. Good geriatric care often requires addressing the

Beware of Unscrupulous Providers

Most of the doctors who focus on geriatrics are not in it for the money, but there is a risk that you could encounter an unscrupulous geriatric practitioner. These doctors run high-volume practices where they see patients very quickly and very superficially. They usually run lots of tests, for a hefty price. If you encounter one of these shady practices, run away as fast as you can.

interactions among problems; multiple visits make addressing those interactions much more challenging.

Geriatric Team Care

Geriatric care is often team care. Geriatricians may use multiple part-
ners to address the breadth of issues. A growing group of health care professionals who are specially qualified to care for older people are geriatric
nurse practitioners. These nurse practitioners (NPs) have had advanced
training in caring for older people. (There is now a special national certifying examination in geriatrics for NPs.) NPs provide care that is almost
identical to that provided by geriatric doctors and generally work with
geriatricians as part of a larger practice team. Because NPs come from a
nursing background, they are often better at talking with patients and
more concerned about the patient as a person. They may be willing and
able to spend more time with older patients. Physician assistants (PAs)
are another fixture of geriatric practice teams, but they usually cannot
provide the same level of independent care as NPs.

Multiple Doctors

Even if your parent or other relative has a geriatrician or a primary
care doctor, chances are they will see a lot of other specialists as well to
treat their various ailments. The average Medicare recipient sees eight
different doctors in the course of a year. This multiplicity of care means
a great deal of confusion and opportunities for mischief. In many cases
one doctor has no idea what the other has done or prescribed. You will
quickly become the best-informed person about your parent's total care.
As such, you need to be a proactive advocate. Ask questions. Bring a full
list of medications to every visit with every doctor and ask each before
they prescribe a new medication to review the list of what the older
person is already taking. If they order a test you think has recently been
performed, say so.

Dealing with Messy Interactions

The primary challenge of geriatric medicine is handling the interactions between different problems. Geriatrics is typically defined as addressing the interaction of multiple problems that often bridge different domains, including medical, emotional, and social. After a certain age, multiple diagnoses are practically guaranteed. The presence of one problem may be complicated by the existence of another. The elderly frequently take multiple medications and they metabolize medications differently than do younger adults. This means they may respond to lower doses and can easily become overmedicated. And unrelated problems can affect treatment. For instance, poor hearing can make it hard to understand doctors' instructions and poor memory can make it hard to remember those directions.

The messy relationships between different problems spill over from the medical world into everyday life. Geriatricians not only have to keep track of their patients' different medical conditions, they have to be clued in to all aspects of their patients' lives. Geriatric illnesses can be exacerbated by different ingredients of an older person's life, and vice versa. For example, if a person has congestive heart failure that causes shortness of breath, and she lives in an apartment on the fourth floor of a building without an elevator, the four sets of stairs she climbs each day will not help her breathe easier. Or if a person has a serious vision problems and a long list of different prescriptions to be taken at different times of the day, the risk of taking the wrong pill skyrockets. Or what if lack of income or mobility prevents an older person from purchasing essential medications or food? And what if an older person is forced to choose between paying for a prescription and paying the rent? Financial resources have a major impact on the ways problems are addressed. The ability to pay for early treatment can delay institutionalization or the need to obtain in-home assistance.

The point is that older people rarely suffer from just one problem. Because older people generally suffer from more than one problem at a time, it may be hard to recognize a new symptom against the background of so much clinical activity. We often compare pinpointing a new symptom in an older patient to discovering a new peak among the Alps. Diagnosing a younger person is more like spotting a skyscraper in the desert. Geriatricians know how to identify that new peak and address it in the context of all the others.

Handling Specialists

Modern medical practice relies heavily on referrals to specialists. Because many older persons have multiple diseases and conditions, they are often treated by several different specialists. Specialties tend to cluster around organs. Most specialists concentrate on one organ system, like the heart or the digestive tract. A cardiopulmonary specialist can tell you exactly what's wrong with a patient's heart but probably is not interested in anything beyond their arteries.

The typical older patient may be seeing four or five different specialists, and multiple specialists can be a risky combination. Specialists can be like teachers assigning homework. Each believes his or her course is the important one. Each one prescribes drugs and establishes a medical regimen to treat one specific problem. They may not consider how their course of treatment will affect anything else. Older people can wind up taking mixtures of medications that interact in dangerous and unforeseen ways. The advice given by one physician may conflict with that of another. You need a traffic cop. You need someone who can put the whole situation into perspective and look for duplications and harmful combinations in the care regimen, who can be sure that all issues and problems are cared for and none are overlooked.

When You Must Be the Traffic Cop

Traditionally, the role of traffic cop is filled by the primary care clinician. But, as explained above, these physicians are in short supply. So family members may find themselves taking on the role of traffic cop for an aging parent. If you start directing care traffic for your parent, you will need to sort through information and look for conflicting recommendations. Though you obviously do not have the medical knowledge to vet medications, you can stand prepared to ask each prescribing physician whether his newest suggestion duplicates or interacts with what is already prescribed. You will need a list of the medications your parent is currently taking because it is very unlikely that the doctor will have one.

Setting Goals

One of the toughest questions facing geriatricians is knowing when a problem is a natural outcome of aging and when it's a symptom of illness. The classic old saw describes an eighty-five-year-old man who complains to his doctor about pain in his right knee. The doctor says, "What can you expect? You're eighty-five." The man responds, "My left knee is eighty-five and it doesn't hurt." The goal of geriatrics is to treat only the things that need treating, and to treat them excellently. But discerning the difference between what is due to aging and what is due to disease is one of the biggest challenges in medicine. Knowing when to treat and when to cope is an art as well as a science. Yes, training and experience play a role, but so do fundamental beliefs. Unfortunately, this means philosophic differences can cramp cooperation between medical and social service professionals. Clinicians and social service workers may have different long-term care goals.

Varying Perspectives Between Clinicians and Social Service Workers

Social service workers view care as filling gaps in a client's ability to cope. They assess a person's daily activities to identify areas of difficulty and then prescribe service packages to address those shortfalls. In the social service world, a good care plan makes up for the client's inabilities.

Clinicians see it differently. They expect to change something as a result of their care plan. The patient should get better—or at least get worse more slowly. Sometimes in geriatric medicine, the goal of good care is simply slowing the rate of decline.

Long-Term Care Requires Collaboration

Because medical caregivers and social service providers may not necessarily share the same goals, they may need to apply more effort toward agreeing on an effective long-term care plan. Caring for older people requires synchronizing the goals of many different people—care professionals, families, and the recipients of care. Long-term care requires genuine collaboration. Identifying shared goals is the first step in this process.

Even if you get past that first step, and reach an agreement on your parent's treatment goals, caring for older adults remains challenging for everyone involved. Professionals and family members alike need to acknowledge that success in caring for older people might not mean finding a cure, it might mean slowing the rate of decline. Changing the clinical trajectory for an older person is a major feat, one that can dramatically improve their quality of life. One may not be able to extend an older person's life span, but one can make that life considerably more pleasant. Long-term care means compromising, consulting, changing goals when conditions change, and complimenting everyone who contributes effectively to an older adult's care. That is the best that can be expected.

Changing Doctors

Even if your parent has had an ongoing relationship with the same doctor, changes to her medical or living situation might disrupt that relationship. For example, if your mother enters a nursing home, her doctor may decide to discontinue treatment. Or a doctor may retire or die. Remember George Burns once quipped that if he knew he was going to live this long he would have gotten a younger doctor.

Doctors and Nursing Homes

When your relative lives in a nursing home the regulations require a primary care doctor of record. For one reason or another, people often change their primary doctor at that time. Some nursing homes require doctors to apply for the privilege of treating patients on-site and to agree to follow rules set by the facility and will not permit the original doctor to practice there. More often, your relative's doctor will not wish to make visits to nursing homes (required at intervals by law) or will not want to go to a nursing home in far-flung locations. Some older people can continue to visit their regular doctor's office, if they are mobile enough and have access to transportation, although most nursing home residents are seen in the facility by the facility doctor. Often the home's medical director cares for the majority of the residents. But more and more physicians are specializing in nursing home care. The medical director has overall responsibility for care in the facility, and even if he or she is not the primary care physician, you can consult that medical director on any matter of concern. Your relative may retain the services of specialists who have seen him or her before; however, if a hospitalization occurs, a new set of doctors may be ushered in depending on where your relative is hospitalized. A nursing home also may have psychologists or mental health consultants, with whom they request or require that you work.

In the best circumstances, the nursing home physicians organize a solid care program and use nurse practitioners to extend their coverage. But all too frequently they have too many patients. Some may make flying visits, swooping in to deal with multiple patients in one visit. As a result, they provide only superficial care. They do only the minimally required paperwork (documentation and writing prescriptions, for example) to meet regulations requiring that each resident be seen monthly. Medicare does not reimburse well for nursing home visits and may refuse to pay a physician for more than one visit a month; so physicians are reluctant to make extra visits to the nursing home. Instead, physicians may opt to handle a problem over the phone, referring the resident to the emergency room if they feel more attention is needed. Sending fragile nursing home residents into stressful emergency room environments should not be a recurring part of a care program.

Getting Assessed

Before making a major change in an older person's long-term care program, such as entering a nursing home, you should schedule a comprehensive geriatric assessment. These assessments serve two purposes: (1) There may be something treatable that could obviate the need for more LTC (generally this is not the case, but it's worth trying). (2) The older person should be in the best shape possible for the transition with the fewest medications needed.

Decisions to admit a person to a nursing home should never be made lightly. Before committing, you should carefully explore other possibilities. Scheduling a geriatric assessment is like scheduling a reality check. The evaluation reviews all problems—both medical and functional. The goal is to size up the person's overall well-being, and determine what supportive services are needed.

Cognitive and physical functioning are tested. These assessments are generally conducted by a team consisting of a geriatrician, a nurse, and a social worker. Other professionals—psychologists, physical and occupational therapists, dentists (even audiologists)—can be brought in if necessary. You can contact the American Geriatrics Society (contact information for the AGS is provided in the appendix) to locate someone nearby who can perform a geriatric assessment. If you do not have access to a private geriatric practice, many academic health centers provide geriatric care evaluations.

Before Choosing Institutional Care

Before deciding that institutional care is necessary, it is worthwhile to see if any of your parent's problems can be corrected. Geriatric assessments are designed to identify and treat any treatable problems. Once the treatable conditions have been dealt with, the geriatric team will help your parent find to ways to cope and to enjoy the best quality of life. This might include therapy, such as physical therapy or occupational therapy for help in performing daily tasks, or it might involve environmental changes that make daily life safer, more supportive, and easier to manage. The chances that a geriatric team will uncover reversible causes of problems like dementia are small. But a geriatric evaluation is still worth the effort. A geriatric team cannot make problems disappear, but they can offer a wide variety of helpful suggestions to make life easier. Besides, a geriatric assessment buys time for considering options and puts you into contact with skilled professionals who can help you make the best choice.

How to Advocate

Getting actively involved in your loved one's care is essential, as is encouraging him or her to be as actively involved as possible. An AARP survey found that people who are more engaged in managing their illness experience fewer problems than those who are less engaged.

Patients Benefit from Being Active in Their Own Care

Compared to the 40 percent of AARP survey respondents who reported being highly and actively involved in their own care, the least active patients:

- Were the most likely to report experiencing problems
- Appeared sicker and had more contact with the health care system than more active respondents
- Were less likely to look out for themselves and less likely to follow their provider's advice than the most active respondents
- And among people with chronic conditions, experiencing a medical error was more likely among less-engaged people.

(AARP Public Policy Institute Beyond 50.09, *Chronic Care: A Call to Action for Health Reform*, Washington, D.C., 2009.)

Ensuring the Best Care Is Up to You

Always bear in mind that long-term care professionals are just that, professionals. They deal with many different patients every day. You should not automatically assume they have your interests closest to heart. While your primary concern is for the relative for whom you care, their primary concern is doing their job. To ensure that your loved one receives the best possible care, you will need to advocate for that care.

The Agency for Healthcare Research and Quality (a federal agency) has prepared some materials designed to help people get better medical care. Below is a series of questions/topics you should raise with a doctor about the care she or he is providing to your loved one and some tips on what you can do to assure that your parent's health care is as good as it can be are offered.

Questions to Ask About Medical Care

1. What is the test for?
2. How many times have you done this?
3. When will I get the results?
4. Why does he need this surgery?
5. Are there any alternatives to surgery?
6. What are the possible complications?
7. Which hospital is best for his needs?
8. How do you spell the name of that drug?
9. Are there any side effects?
10. Will this medicine interact with medicines that he's already taking?

Source: Agency for Healthcare Research and Quality.

Steps You Can Take to Be Involved in Your Loved One's Health Care

The single most important way you can help to prevent errors is to get your loved one involved in his or her own care.

That means he or she should take part in every decision about his or her health care. Research shows that patients who are more involved with their care tend to get better results. Some specific tips, based on the latest scientific evidence about what works best, follow.

Medicines

1. Make sure that all of your loved one's doctors know about everything they are taking. This includes prescription and over-the-counter medicines, and dietary supplements such as vitamins and herbs.

2. At least once a year, bring all of the patient's medicines and supplements with you to his or her doctor. "Brown bagging" one's medicines can help foster discussion about them and find out if there are any problems. It can also help the doctor keep your loved one's records up to date, which can help you get better-quality care. (But you should also keep a careful record of every medication.)

3. Make sure the doctor knows about any allergies and adverse reactions your loved one has had to medicines. This can help him or her avoid getting a medicine that could be harmful.

4. When the doctor writes a prescription, make sure you and the patient can read it. If you can't read the doctor's handwriting, the pharmacist might not be able to either.

5. Ask for information about medicines in terms you can understand—both when medicines are prescribed and when the patient receives them.

   • What is the medicine for?

   • How is he or she supposed to take it, and for how long?

- What side effects are likely? What do I do if they occur?
- Is this medicine safe to take with other medicines or dietary supplements I am taking?
- What food, drink, or activities should I avoid while taking this medicine?

6. When you pick up your medicine from the pharmacy, ask: Is this the medicine that my doctor prescribed?

   A study by the Massachusetts College of Pharmacy and Allied Health Sciences found that 88 percent of medicine errors involved the wrong drug or the wrong dose.

7. If you have any questions about the directions on your medicine labels, ask.

   Medicine labels can be hard to understand. For example, ask if "four doses daily" means taking a dose every six hours around the clock or just during regular waking hours.

8. Ask your pharmacist for the best device to measure your liquid medicine. Also, ask questions if you're not sure how to use it.

   Research shows that many people do not understand the right way to measure liquid medicines. For example, many use household teaspoons, which often do not hold a true teaspoon of liquid. Special devices, like marked syringes, help people to measure the right dose. Being told how to use the devices helps even more.

9. Ask for written information about the side effects your medicine could cause.

If you know what might happen, you will be better prepared if it does—or, if something unexpected happens instead. That way, you can report the problem right away and get help before it gets worse. A study found that written information about medicines can help patients recognize problem side effects and then give that information to their doctor or pharmacist.

Hospital Stays

1. If you have a choice, choose a hospital at which many patients have the procedure or surgery you need.

   Research shows that patients tend to have better results when they are treated in hospitals that have a great deal of experience with their condition.

2. If you are in a hospital, consider asking all health care workers who have direct contact with you whether they have washed their hands.

   Hand washing is an important way to prevent the spread of infections in hospitals. Yet it is not done regularly or thoroughly enough. A recent study found that when patients checked whether health care workers washed their hands, the workers washed their hands more often and used more soap.

3. When you are being discharged from the hospital, ask your doctor to explain the treatment plan you will use at home.

   This includes learning about your medicines and finding out when you can get back to your regular activities. Research shows that at discharge time, doctors think their patients understand more than they really do about what they should or should not do when they return home.

Surgery

1. If you are having surgery, make sure that you, your doctor, and your surgeon all agree and are clear on exactly what will be done.

   Doing surgery at the wrong site (for example, operating on the left knee instead of the right) is rare. But even once is too often. The good news is that wrong-site surgery is 100 percent preventable. The American Academy of Orthopaedic Surgeons urges its members to sign their initials directly on the site to be operated on before the surgery.

Other Steps You Can Take[11]

1. Speak up if you have questions or concerns.

    You have a right to question anyone who is involved with your care.

2. Make sure that someone, such as your personal doctor, is in charge of your care.

    This is especially important if you have many health problems or are in a hospital.

3. Make sure that all health professionals involved in your care have important health information about you.

    Do not assume that everyone knows everything they need to.

4. Ask a family member or friend to be there with you and to be your advocate (someone who can help get things done and speak up for you if you can't).

    Even if you think you don't need help now, you might need it later.

5. Know that "more" is not always better.

    It is a good idea to find out why a test or treatment is needed and how it can help you. You could be better off without it.

6. If you have a test, don't assume that no news is good news. Ask about the results.

7. Learn about your condition and treatments by asking your doctor and nurse and by using other reliable sources.

For example, treatment recommendations based on the latest scientific evidence are available from the National Guideline Clearinghouse at www.guideline.gov. Ask your doctor if your treatment is based on the latest evidence.

---

11. Source: ahrq.gov/questionsaretheanswer.

Managing Transitions

The most dangerous time in medical care is when a patient moves from one care system to another; for example, hospital discharges or being sent to the emergency room. All sorts of bad things can happen at those hand-offs. Critical information is lost or distorted. It is a time for hypervigilance.

An AARP survey found that older people with chronic conditions and their caregivers expressed many concerns about transitions from hospitals and other health care facilities. Overall, transitions were stressful and created many communication and other issues.

The most frequently mentioned issues were:
* Loss of mobility and/or independence
* Uncertain expectations for recovery and/or prognosis
* Pain
* Anxiety
* Not remembering their doctor's instructions
* Feeling abandoned

The most frequently mentioned issues for caregivers were:
* Finding resources, such as medical equipment and services
* Arranging for assistance in and around the home, both paid and unpaid
* Communicating with doctors and other health professionals
* Finances/affordability
* Uncertain expectations for their relative's or friend's recovery and/or prognosis
* Managing their relative's or friend's expectations
* Not enough time for competing demands (e.g., care coordination, job, children, self)
* Stress/emotional strain/guilt

(AARP Public Policy Institute Beyond 50.09, *Chronic Care: A Call to Action for Health Reform*, Washington, D.C., 2009, www.aarp.org/research/ppi/health-care/health-qual/articles/beyond)

Hiring a Case Manager

You can be your parent's advocate or you can hire the services of a professional advocate. There are no easy long-term care decisions. If you are unsure about your ability to work your way through a complicated system (and few laypeople have the experience and emotional stamina for this task), it may pay to hire a case manager. Your case manager can set realistic care goals and protect your interests (see the section on Geriatric Care Managers in Chapter Ten for more information).

Family as Case Manager

If you decide not to hire a case manager, then you should be prepared to take on that role. Acting as a case manager means going above and beyond being a caregiver. You must keep track of doctors and drugs. We want to believe that doctors' records are readily accessible and contain all the relevant information. Unfortunately, that's not always the case. It's better to be proactive. Remind doctors about existing diagnoses and medications. Each time a new drug is prescribed, ask the doctor if it duplicates or interferes with any other drug in your care recipient's regime. Pharmacists also can provide expert advice to help you avoid medication mix-ups. Talking to the doctor and pharmacist is useless, however, if you do not have an up-to-date medication list.

Table 3.1: Medication List

Medication	Reason for drug	Dosage	Frequency (how often per day, when)	Doctor who prescribed it	Date of last prescription

MANAGING MEDICATIONS

When a medication is prescribed, you want to get used to asking how long and for what purpose. After a period of time at another visit you may ask about blood levels. Have the blood levels been checked to be sure they are still at a therapeutic range? There were more than a few times over the course of my mother's illness where her anti-seizure medicine blood levels would not have been checked had we not reminded the lab technician, who went and checked with the doctor before drawing blood to be sure that it was needed (it was in all instances).

It is easy to get confused about medications because they often have a different name from what you are used to. You need to specifically ask the doctor and the pharmacist: "My mother's anti-seizure medication was prescribed as 'X' [name], but this says 'Y' [name]. Is that the same thing and should the dosage and frequency be the same?" Also ask if the new drug interacts with any of her other medications—the pharmacist will likely be the most up to date on this, but the doctor should too. OFTEN the doctor will not know all the medications your loved one is on unless you bring the current list of medications to the examining room at the time of the visit.   —DEB PAONE, CAREGIVING DAUGHTER

You should create and update a medication record that lists each medication—prescribed and over-the-counter, vitamins, herbals, and other supplements—that your parent is taking. Table 3.1 can be used as a model for a medication list.

Drug Details You Should Record

Information about each medication, like what pharmacy it comes from, when to take it, whether it can be mixed with alcohol, and whether it should be taken with or without food can also be essential. It is best to use the same pharmacy for all medications. This increases your pharmacist's ability to keep track of the drugs prescribed and identify potential interactions or duplications. Some pharmacists have access to computer programs to do just that.

You should also keep a list of all the doctors your parent visits. Table 3.2 provides a basic format for such a list.

Table 3.2: Doctor List

Doctor's name	Specialty	Address	Phone number	Name of office assistant	Date of last visit

Preparing for Doctor's Visits

The medical care system is not user friendly. In many cases, technology is substituted for personal contact. Doctors are under great pressure to see as many patients as possible. That usually means brief encounters. The average physician visit lasts twelve minutes. That is not enough time to explain any changes or to review ongoing problems. Twelve minutes is not enough time to give or receive information. With visits that short, you need to be efficient. Physicians don't structure visits well; that task falls to you. So you've got to be prepared.

One way to prepare for each visit is to make a list of questions and observations. You should actually write these questions down in advance of the visit. You may even want to rehearse the visit in advance.

Questions and Considerations to Record Before and During Your Parent's Doctor Visits

1. What is your number one priority for today's visit?
2. Has anything unusual happened or have you noticed a gradual but concerning change?
3. Has a new symptom developed or has there been a change in behavior?
4. If a new medication is prescribed, show the doctor the list of all the medications currently being taken.

5. Can any medications be eliminated? Is there risk of interactions with those already prescribed?

6. Are there any possibilities to save money by substituting generic medications for brand name drugs?

You should have a problem list where you record every diagnosis or significant problem your parent has, and when and how it was last treated. Table 3.3 shows a simple way to make that list.

Table 3.3: Diagnosis List

Diagnosis/ problem	Name of doctor treating it	Date of last visit	Medications prescribed for it

Making the Most of the Appointment

You may feel rushed, but it is vital, if you are acting as your parent's advocate, that you speak with the doctor about all the necessary issues, and that you and your parent understand the doctor's instructions. Some doctors have a bad habit of speaking with their backs to their clients or giving critical information as they are walking out the door. Be polite but be firm. You came prepared; you should leave informed. If you do not understand something, ask the doctor to explain it again. If you have to ask more than once, do it.

Understanding the doctor's instructions means believing that they are reasonable. If the doctor prescribes a medicine the patient cannot afford or will not take, it is a waste of everyone's time. Leaving the doctor's office with an unclear picture of what is expected is dangerous. At the end of the visit, you can negotiate with the doctor. You can trade recommendations, check to make sure that you both have realistic plans and goals, and make sure you're both on the same page. Both of you may

Make Sure the Patient Has Her Own Voice

Because doctors try to see as many patients a day as possible, they will try to keep the visit as brief as possible. In order to do that, they often communicate with the most articulate person in the room, usually a family member. If you are the caregiving family member in this position, be alert to the possibility that the older patient may be bypassed or ignored. This is degrading to the patient and reduces their independence. Try to redirect the doctor's questions and recommendations to the older patient.

need to make compromises. The key is to make sure you set a plan you can both live with.

A Proactive Approach to Chronic Illness

In a perfect world, doctors would instruct patients with chronic illnesses and their families to make regular and systematic observations about their conditions and report any early signs of change. In this world, few doctors do. The current fee-for-service system does not make it rewarding for physicians to monitor a patient's status outside of an office visit. But that's no excuse for not taking a proactive approach to dealing with chronic illnesses. You can take on the task of monitoring your parent's condition. For many common problems, it is not hard to imagine what you should be recording. Keeping careful records is the best way to manage chronic illnesses. This way, you will detect early signs of deterioration and be able to rapidly notify clinicians.

An early intervention can prevent severe complications. This approach requires teamwork between you and a clinician. Observing and recording your parent's status doesn't help unless you have a clinician who is prepared to react promptly. The best you might hope for is to undertake the monitoring and make an arrangement with a physician that he or she will respond quickly to a call for help. A good monitoring arrangement will include tracking essential variables and agreeing on what counts as an early warning of potential problems.

Many kinds of observations must be made to track the progress of a disease. The observations should be recorded on paper daily and brought in with each visit and shown to the doctor. These observations provide the doctor with a pattern of problems that reflect the progression of the disease. You should bring all of your lists—diagnoses, medications, and ongoing observations—to every doctor and emergency room visit. Here is a list of conditions and observations your loved one's doctors will need to be aware of during appointments:

Examples of Conditions Where Self-Observation and Reporting Can Be Useful

PROBLEM	OBSERVATION
Diabetes	Blood sugar
Congestive heart failure	Weight Edema Shortness of breath
Angina	Episodes of chest pain
Hypertension	Blood pressure
Chronic Obstructive Pulmonary Disease	Need for extra inhalers Exercise tolerance
Asthma	Peak flow
Falls	History of new falls and circumstances
Dementia	Independence Memory Wandering

How to Talk with a Doctor

Sometimes communication between patients, their families, and their doctors can become tense, or even angry. It is important to remember that fighting with the doctor is not productive. In most cases, you should trust the doctor's years of medical school and experience. They probably do know what is best for the older person. But they may not always be well versed in geriatrics.

But what if you have found a miracle cure? The media is full of articles about medical breakthroughs. If you are an active, involved caregiver, you are probably very aware of new developments that could affect your parent. So you may have seen more about a new drug or treatment than the doctor. Even if you believe you have found an amazing solution, you need to broach the subject of a new cure carefully. Most doctors are rightfully skeptical about announcements of wonder cures, especially when they've been hyped by the media. And doctors are only human. No one likes to feel uninformed or one-upped, especially when their professional pride is on the line. If you do decide to talk with your doctor about a cure or treatment, be polite. If they shoot you down, feel free to ask for reasons. But do not become belligerent. If they say no and stick to it, you should accept their answer. If you are still convinced there is a better way to treat the problem, find another doctor who is more sympathetic, or at least seek a second opinion.

Health Insurance Portability and Accountability Act

Even if you usually agree with the doctor, federal regulations can make communication unnecessarily complicated. Parts of the Health Insurance Portability and Accountability Act (HIPAA) were designed to protect medical records from prying eyes. In reality, they've done more to complicate care than to protect privacy. Care providers often misinterpret the law, and refuse to release any information without written authorization. This can have catastrophic consequences. If the patient is confused or suffering from dementia, they cannot necessarily give the informed consent necessary to release information. As a caregiver, you should be sure to have a signed (and, if possible, notarized) statement authorizing your access to all medical data. If you take on the job of coordinating care, make sure you are properly equipped.

Keeping Records

In addition to keeping lists of medications, diagnoses, and benchmarks of different conditions, you should establish a special place to keep all pertinent information about your loved one. These would include:

- Social Security number
- Medicare number
- Medicaid number (if appropriate)
- VA number (if appropriate)
- Supplemental health insurance policy numbers (and contact phone numbers)
- Long-term care insurance number
- Medication list
- Diagnosis list
- Doctor list (with phone numbers)
- Advance directives
- Copy of the will
- Special bequests or requests
- List of all bank accounts
- Safe deposit keys
- List of all investments (including real estate)
- Insurance information: life insurance company and policy numbers, car insurance, business insurance
- List of monthly bill companies
- Phone numbers of persons to call in case of a problem (e.g., building manager, next-door neighbor)

Being Informed

Nowadays it is easy to be informed. It is harder to be well informed. The media is filled with stories about the latest medical breakthrough. Sometimes this hype is justified; sometimes it is not.

Whatever your disdain for the media, it is now possible to learn a great deal about almost any syndrome or disease by going online. Skillful practitioners of Web-based legerdemain can uncover a huge treasure trove of information. The hard part is distinguishing what is true. Many physicians are put off by patients or family members who come to the office armed with printouts and facts. Sometimes they are right to be annoyed because the quality of data is poor and misleading.

But many times, the information a website provides is solid. There are good websites; I've listed some of my favorites in the appendix. You can look up various topics of interest and get a sense of the degree of coherence in what is said. So do not be afraid to look for information and do not be afraid to tell (or ask) the doctor about what you have found. While some doctors are peeved when a family member raises a study that contradicts his recommendations, most will respond with seriousness and forbearance.

Chapter Three—Points to Ponder

Aging complicates diagnoses. It is often hard to distinguish what is due to aging from what is disease.

Aging specialists (geriatricians) are rare. Even informed primary care doctors may be hard to find.

Medical regimens are complex. Most older people see many doctors and hence may have confusing medical regimens, with great potential for mischief and duplications.

Caregivers are traffic cops. They must be well informed.

Record-keeping is critical. Keep good, up-to-date records of diagnoses, doctors, and medications.

Track symptoms, especially changes. If an older person's condition is changing, seek help.

Be prepared for every doctor visit. Decide in advance what you want to accomplish.

Feel empowered. If you have seen something that might help your parent, ask about it. If something seems inconsistent, ask about it.

Confirm doctor's orders. Make sure you understand what the doctor has recommended and that the plan seems realistic.

Four

Caring for Yourself

A caregiver who does not care for herself cannot care well for anyone else. There is no perfect solution to the reality that caregiving for an elderly loved one can be an all-consuming responsibility with inordinate demands, leaving you with very little time or resources to really take care of yourself the way you should. Nonetheless, don't let go of the effort to keep yourself healthy and well in the face of the physical and emotional challenges of caregiving. It is well worth the investment of time and creative energy to find workable solutions to your own need for a nutritious diet, adequate sleep, and regular physical exercise. Other caregivers have walked in your shoes, and can provide incredibly helpful ideas for how to keep yourself going when the going gets rough.

Caregivers are by their very definition giving profoundly of themselves. The rewards are immeasurable. And equally immeasurable are the stresses. Caregivers must know their limits. Caregiving is hard work and can even be dangerous. It needs and deserves ongoing and at times intense support. Too often caregivers see themselves as indispensable. And they are indispensable, but they are not immortal. They're convinced that no one can deliver care the way they do. They might be right, but acting on those convictions is not realistic. Caregivers need help. You need a break. You will last longer and be able to do a better job every day if you get a little relief.

A TOTAL COMMITMENT

Exercise really helps with stamina, but I was not always able to go to the fitness center on a regular schedule when I was caring for my mother. I had to find small ways to add in exercise, like doing some stretches while cooking, parking farther away from the store entrance, taking the stairs when possible, getting ankle weights and walking around the house with them. Having a dog to walk every morning (no fenced-in backyard) meant that I had to have at least twenty minutes where I'd be outside and walking. If possible, set a date and time for exercise in your calendar and keep to it.

My nutritional status definitely suffered during the years of caregiving. Time and energy were the two biggest hurdles. Again, I did not always follow my own better judgment. I was good at eating a decent breakfast (every morning protein, carbs, and fruit—no sweets!) and something reasonable midday. Dinner was difficult, both in terms of timing and energy to prepare. (The end of the day when you are sitting on the sofa and reach for the TV remote is the most dangerous time of the day in terms of nutritional status.) When caregiving needs are great, this is not the time to fuss. So many options now exist for grab-and-go meals at grocery stores that are very healthy. Buy a supply at the beginning of the week, add fresh greens and fruit, and forget cooking unless it's something simple like frozen pasta and vegetable dinners that you make in one pot (the only downside is the sodium content, which you can "dilute" by adding more uncooked frozen vegetables to the whole pot—they never give you enough anyway). An additional suggestion is to make a big pot or dish of something on the weekend (e.g., chili, baked chicken and rice, Crock-Pot stew, meatballs) and have it in various ways all week.

—DEB PAONE, CAREGIVING DAUGHTER

Pace Yourself

Caregiving is stressful. Taking breaks is not selfish; it is self-preservation, for you and your parent. If you are constantly exhausted, it is not good for whomever you're caring for, and it's certainly not good for you. Caregivers are more prone to develop illnesses of their own, especially as they age. They are likely to suffer bouts of depression. Most caregivers rate their health lower than non-caregivers. As a caregiver, you need to pace yourself like a distance runner, not a sprinter. Everyone suffers if the caregiver collapses. Too often there is no one to hand the baton to and the older person is forced into an institution.

THE HONOR OF CAREGIVING

Sometimes it wasn't pretty—the home-care nurse canceling because of a snowstorm, the weekends devoted to parents rather than to the stuff of our own lives sometimes resented, workloads among siblings appearing uneven, worry about our mother and what might happen when we couldn't be there. . . . But we made it. Dad didn't actually die in his beloved home but in the local hospital after a two-day stay, with his wife of sixty-four years and his children at his bedside, holding his hand. We all felt a sense of victory. Victory for a long life well-lived, for our ability to help Dad realize his fondest wish to never have to move from his farm home. But victory also for being able to give back, in the most intimate sense, some of the loving care with which we had been raised, for strength of character in caregiving we didn't know we had, for the bond reinforced in our family, that together, we were a force to reckoned with. Memories of the caregiving struggles we had all experienced gave way to a sense of having done it right, of having given honor to our parents and to who they raised us to be. This caregiving was one of the best things I have done in my life.

—GAYLE KVENVOLD, CAREGIVING DAUGHTER

Many Forms of Support

Different caregivers need different kinds of help. Fortunately, caregiver support comes in many forms. There are support groups for caregivers that offer emotional support and reassurance, often from peers experiencing the same stresses. There are various forms of respite care, which allows you to take a much-needed break from caregiving (more information on respite care is available in the Respite Care section of Chapter Ten). And there is training to help you be a more successful caregiver and cope with problems you will most likely encounter as a caregiver.

PREPARE FOR THE MARATHON, NOT THE SPRINT

For caregivers of those with diagnoses that are likely to last years versus months or weeks, the first advice I can give is to orient yourself to the reality that this is going to be a long haul. This means that you will need to figure out how to continue to eat, sleep, work, and hopefully exercise and occasionally socialize in the midst of what is going on with the person you love and who has needs. This sounds simple, but it's not, and sometimes you have to make a difficult decision between your own basic needs and the person's wishes for more of you. *These are the times to ask for help.* Sometimes there is no good solution as you are pulled between your family and work responsibilities, yourself, and your loved one who is ill. In these cases any choice may bring guilt. Let go of guilt because in the long run it takes more energy away from you that is not available later when you really need it.

—DEB PAONE, CAREGIVING DAUGHTER

TALK TO SOMEONE

It is a lonely job full of emotional ups and downs. Your immediate family members are also going through the experience and have their own burdens. They may not be able to listen to your pain or help you carry your burden. There may be others, such as through your faith community, with whom you can share a bit of what's going on and how it affects you.

—DEB PAONE, CAREGIVING DAUGHTER

Table 4.1 lists a number of questions that can help point out when caregivers are at risk and need some help. The scale that comes from these questions has been used to identify caregivers at risk and to successfully intervene.

Table 4.1: Dementia-Caregiver Self-Appraisal Scale (CR = care recipient)

1.	Do you have written information about memory loss, Alzheimer's disease, or dementia?
2.	Can CR get to dangerous objects (e.g., gun, knife, or other sharp objects)?
3.	Do you ever leave CR alone or unsupervised in the home?
4.	Does CR try to leave the home and wander outside?
5.	Does CR drive?
6.	Overall, how satisfied have you been in the past month with the help you have received from family members, friends, or neighbors?
7.	In the past month, have you had trouble falling asleep, staying asleep, or waking up too early in the morning?
8.	In the past month, how satisfied have you been with the support, comfort, interest, and concern you have received from others?
9.	In general, would you say your health is: *Excellent* *Very good* *Good* *Fair* *Poor*
10.	During the past week, I felt depressed: *Rarely or none of the time* (less than 1 day) *Some or a little of the time* (1 to 2 days) *Occasionally or a moderate amount of the time* (3 to 4 days) *Most or almost all of the time* (5 to 7 days)
11.	How often in the past six months have you felt like screaming or yelling at CR because of the way he or she behaved? *Never* *Sometimes* *Often* *Always*
12.	How often in the past six months, have you had to keep yourself from hitting or slapping CR because of the way he or she behaved? *Never* *Sometimes* *Often* *Always*

Table 4.1 (continued)

13.	Do you feel stressed between caring for CR and trying to meet other responsibilities (work/family)? *Never* *Rarely* *Sometimes* *Often* *Nearly always*
14.	Do you feel strained when you are around CR? *Never* *Rarely* *Sometimes* *Often* *Nearly always*
15.	Is it hard or stressful for you to help CR in basic daily activities, like bathing, changing clothes, brushing teeth, or shaving? *Never* *Rarely* *Sometimes* *Often* *Nearly always*
16.	Providing help to CR has made me feel good about myself. *Disagree a lot* *Disagree a little* *Neither agree nor disagree* *Agree a little* *Agree a lot*

Source: S. J. Czaja, L. N. Gitlin, R. Schulz, et al. "Development of the Risk Appraisal Measure: A Brief Screen to Identify Risk Areas and Guide Interventions for Dementia Caregivers," *Journal of the American Geriatrics Society* 57, no. 6 (June 2009):1064–72.

Guilt, Anger, and Depression

Giving care involves a lot of mixed emotions. You will inevitably feel guilty and angry, and even more guilty for feeling angry. You probably never thought you could wish that the person you are caring for was dead. But you will. Hugh Marriott's whimsical book *The Selfish Pig's Guide to Caring*, about his own caregiving experience and the emotions it generated, is a good source of reassurance that your feelings are not unique or inhumane.

Be Realistic

You need to be realistic. You will never do enough. It is not in the nature of caring to ever hope to reach that goal. Even more frustrating, the person receiving the care may be incapable of expressing gratitude either because she is too confused to appreciate what is being done or is truly not appreciative.

Whether you call it "burnout" or "compassionate fatigue," you are going to crash at some point. The goal is to minimize the fallout and preserve the caregiving structure. The alternative is an institution.

Institutions Are Not Failure

At the same time, it is important to recognize that putting a loved one in a nursing home is not a hallmark of caregiving failure. Some people may be better off in such a setting. Certainly removing much of the stress of caring from the family may make the visits more enjoyable and bearable. One person commented that putting her father in a nursing home freed up the family to be a family. Visits became more pleasurable. She no longer had to worry about his clinical status and she could just visit.

Separation Anxiety

Even with the many support options available to caretakers, those who most need such support often stubbornly refuse to accept help. They have convinced themselves that their care is the only care that will work. While this is very understandable, this attitude obviously makes it very hard to offer them any respite, and everyone needs some time away from such a stressful task. Caregiver burnout ultimately harms both the caregiver and the patient. Some organizations, like the Alzheimer's Association, have developed creative ways to circumvent this dilemma. One option is to combine caregivers' support with day care. The Alzheimer's patients attend day care while their caregivers attend a support group and even get some free time, although it is not clear that all caregivers given some time off would prefer to spend it in a support group.

Anxious caregivers can become even more unwilling to use respite care if their loved one seems unhappy to be left in the care of a new person. If a caregiver is already reluctant to use respite care, he or she may use a rocky start as justification to call the whole thing off. Ultimately, this is the wrong approach. Caregivers need to recognize their care recipient's reaction for what it truly is: separation anxiety. Of course your beloved older person is more comfortable having you around, but that doesn't mean using respite care is a bad idea. It just requires an adjustment period. Just like you wouldn't let your child drop out of school if she cried on the first day, you should not abandon the idea of respite care because your older person is not initially pleased to be cared for by someone new.

Support Groups

Some people find relief in support groups; others do not. They come in many forms. Some are organized by disease, such as Alzheimer's disease. Some involve meeting together, and hence raise logistical issues about who will take care of the care recipient while you are attending, therefore some are run in conjunction with day care. Others are organized online, often simply as chat rooms.

The idea of spending your limited free time listening to yourself and others share stories about how hard your lives are may not seem appealing. But you might find comfort in knowing your situation is not unique. You can also swap valuable tips on how to cope with the challenges of caregiving. Support groups can help you learn how to protect yourself from the everyday stress of caregiving. You will find personal, real-life strategies on how to keep healthy, and how to safely meet your loved one's needs. Some support groups even run patient-care training sessions.

Training

Most caregivers find practical advice more helpful than just support, but they are not mutually exclusive. Training for caregivers tends to focus on how to be a better, more successful, and less stressed caregiver. It is especially helpful if you are caring for a parent with dementia, because it can address how to deal with behavior problems and how to cope with the various stages as the dementia worsens. Most training takes place in group settings, but a growing supply of training materials is available online. And of course, there are lots of books on this topic. I have included a list of some of my favorites in the appendix.

Finding Time for Fun

You will not make it if you do not take regular breaks. These respites need to be more than getting some badly needed sleep. You need to identify what you can do to derive active pleasure. You deserve to reward yourself. For some people, that may be a lavish vacation or a fancy meal. For others, it may just be going to a movie with friends. Know yourself. Indulge yourself a little. It will help you and the person you are caring for.

Try to plan regular opportunities to get away even for a few hours. Most people get more from these breaks if they involve interacting with others, but some need time alone. You know yourself. Meals with friends or going to a movie are a good idea. Make a firm date. Sometimes a crisis will intervene, but be sure it is a real crisis and not an excuse to cancel. Movies are better than plays because they can be scheduled more flexibly.

The Tipping Point

If you have taken on the task of caring for a loved one, it is important to acknowledge upfront that the informal family care system eventually runs out of steam. There are some things you can do to delay that point of collapse, but there will come a time when you will not be able to be your loved one's sole provider of care (more information on the tipping point is available in the Calling for Help section in Chapter Nine). Learning personal-care skills and coping skills can help. So can getting help and sharing the load with others. Taking advantage of caregiver training and offers for relief from the strain of caregiving will allow you to balance your own needs while giving effective care for as long as possible.

GIVE YOURSELF A BREAK

Every now and then you may need to plan some kind of trip (even for a day) where you physically get away and try to renew your energy. There was a retreat center and a spa about a thirty-minute drive from home that I used several times over the course of the three-plus years. One night with a full day following was a welcome respite from everything.

—DEB PAONE, CAREGIVING DAUGHTER

Chapter Four—Points to Ponder

Consider some form of group therapy. It can be an in-person caregivers' group or an informal network. There are lots of such organizations on the Web. Or you might just want to join an online chat room of others in a similar situation.

Take care of your own health. Do not ignore little problems.

Recognize the signs of depression and get help. They include fatigue, trouble sleeping, change in appetite (both too little or too much), loss of interest in things, and generalized anxiety, as well as just feeling sad.

Five

Daily Life

As your parent ages and becomes less independent and more in need of various forms of caregiving—whether from you or from others—the shape and texture of her daily life will change. At first, these changes will feel subtle and gradual, and if both of your parents are still alive and living together, they may develop rituals of compensation and interdependence that all but mask their individual frailties. For example, if Dad's hearing is deteriorating rapidly, but Mom tends to translate for him, they may get on more or less fine. But eventually, changes may come that alter your parent's ability to function in ways that can no longer be minimized or overlooked. Examples include changes in a parent's ability to drive, eat independently, and look after the care and grooming of her own body or home, for example. At these times, it is essential that you recognize the changes that are occurring and have the courage and skill to respond appropriately.

Driving

As people age, they cannot safely continue many of their hobbies and activities. One of the hardest things for many old people to lose is their license to drive. However, there will come a point where it is no longer safe for an older person to drive. Having car keys represents a major milestone going up and coming down. In American society, the right to drive is a major symbol of autonomy. Teenagers all long for the moment they can get behind the wheel. Older people dread the moment when they are dragged away from that same wheel. Even when simple calculations show that maintaining a vehicle is uneconomical, its value transcends mere money. It is the symbol of independence, and its loss cannot be exaggerated.

Loss of safe driving ability can be the result of many different factors. Vision problems are a common cause. Cataracts can cause glares and halos that make night driving difficult and dangerous, but they are readily correctable by surgery. But older drivers with macular denegation (the loss of central vision) literally cannot see what is in front of them. And glaucoma (the loss of peripheral vision) can make perceiving pedestrians and cars turning right or left difficult or impossible. Aside from vision-related problems, older drivers with dementia are likely to get lost, or react poorly in crises. Drivers with dementia are almost twice as likely to have a car crash compared to those without it. There is general agreement that persons with moderately severe dementia should not drive. Most of these conditions come on gradually. But eventually the impairment will reach an unsafe level, and it will be time to hand over the car keys. This is often a very difficult situation to manage well.

There are formal assessments (including real and simulated road tests) to ascertain an older person's abilities to drive and respond to emer-

My eighty-eight-year-old friend, Liz, called me on the phone one day. She wanted to go shopping for a new car. Her niece had a new Yaris, and Liz loved that car. At the age when most people no longer drive, Liz was buying a new car! What optimism! Unfortunately, she got a speeding ticket when she passed a patrolman on a state highway at six in the morning.

—JOANN HOWITZ, CAREGIVER AND PHYSICAL THERAPIST

gency situations. A driver rehabilitation specialist can evaluate a person's suitability to drive.

Denial of Driving Danger

Usually family members will recognize the driving danger first. Denial on the part of the older person is common. Older people will insist that they are still perfectly capable of driving. They rationalize that they drive only in familiar areas (as if the other drivers are familiar, too). They drive very slowly (and drive everyone else crazy). Coaxing your loved one into hanging up the keys will be difficult. In contemporary society, the loss of a driver's license is a social catastrophe. It makes little difference whether one relinquishes the privilege of driving voluntarily or if it is taken away by a doctor or the DMV. Not driving means a major loss of both status and autonomy. Transportation falls into the hands of others, both paid and unpaid. People argue that taking taxis is cheaper than maintaining a car, but doing this usually falls flat. On top of higher costs, each trip by taxi has to be planned. Spontaneity and independence are seriously cut down. In rural areas, public transportation may be extremely limited or nonexistent.

Avoid Subterfuge

Some experts recommend various devious strategies like hiding car keys, or filing them down so they no longer work, disabling the vehicle, or sending the car out for "repairs" only to have it never return, or selling it outright. In general, it is better to try to avoid subterfuge. Devious strategies for taking away the car keys can be destructive. Especially when dementia is involved, family members may resort to lying when reasoning fails. They invent complicated stories about why the car is no longer working or is being impounded. These tangled webs are difficult to keep up. People with dementia may have faulty memories, but they are not stupid. Inconsistencies will appear. It may be more effective to couch

COPING AFTER DRIVING IS OVER

Once my mother gave up driving there were four options open to her for getting around. The first was a volunteer ride program that she was able to use once a week. The second was friends and neighbors. Third, me, and fourth, taxis. Other programs offered promises for help that did not materialize, such as transportation offered by the local cancer society or the local health care system. The problem with taxis was not just the cost, but the worry about whether the driver would help her up and down stairs and into the building once she got where she was headed. Friends turned out to be the most reliable option, and I filled in where I could.   —DEBORAH PAONE, CAREGIVING DAUGHTER

FAKING A BROKEN CAR

One family described the simple but sly method they used to get an older parent with dementia to stop driving. They removed the distributor cap so that the car would not start. They convinced their father that the car could not be repaired and had it towed away. This strategy may have been effective, but is not recommended.

suggestions in terms of helping you (e.g., by relieving your anxiety and worry) than to focus on the older person being at risk.

Choose the Right Messenger

One helpful strategy is to have someone outside the family deliver the message. Professionals can be very convincing. Most older people today have a lot of respect for physicians. A physician, preferably one who knows the older driver well, can make a solid case for stopping driving. He can even write a prescription for not driving. Blaming it on a specific disease, rather than simply old age, can make the case more persuasive and palatable.

My father-in-law had macular degeneration but kept driving. Despite our repeated suggestions that he give up driving, he drove very slowly and usually only in familiar areas. (There is some weird belief that you will hit fewer obstacles in familiar territory.) He went for his regular check-up with his ophthalmologist, who asked him how he had gotten there. When he said he had driven himself, the doctor asked for his keys and said he would drive the car home after work. My father-in-law never drove again. Would that there were more doctors like that! Unfortunately, I know of few doctors so committed to their patients' well-being as to take that step. The task typically falls to the family, and they have much less clout.

By contrast, my mother, who was showing early signs of dementia, was increasingly getting lost. One day she had a minor accident, and we suggested that maybe this was a good time to sell her car. To our astonishment she readily acquiesced.

Other potentially influential figures, including clergy or highly re-spected family friends, may be able to persuasively add the weight of their opinions.

Another solution is to report the older person to the Department of Motor Vehicles, which may then request a formal test of driving skills.

Eating: Nutrition, Taste, Safety, and Pleasure

For everyone, the simple act of eating represents myriad complex expectations, from pleasure to autonomy to variety, independence, and even self-expression. For many people, this is also true of cooking and food selection and preparation, even if it is as simple as pouring cereal from a box or toasting bread. These simple acts of self-care tend to be much more significant than simple self-sustenance. Unfortunately, aging tends to complicate the process of food selection, preparation, and con-sumption in a variety of ways that are physical, emotional, and logistical. Caregivers must watch for and know when to respond to changes in eat-ing patterns in their loved one.

MAINTAINING NORMALITY AND JOY IN COOKING AND EATING

Cooking was one of the abilities that diminished rapidly for my mother early on in the course of her illness. Therefore I would buy extra ingredients and take some to my mom to make her home-cooked meals on the weekend while we visited together. She was then able to feel part of the cooking and meal-planning process, which helped her "feel more normal." Make sure you invest in small freezer-quality containers that can be taken out and slipped into the microwave as is. My mother resisted/refused Meals On Wheels and a home-delivered shopping/grocery service. She also tried and then did not renew a service that brought already made meals to her home on a weekly basis.

—DEB PAONE, CAREGIVING DAUGHTER

But just because Dad has stopped asking for seconds of everything does not mean you need to worry. Healthy eating is important at all ages, but many older people will have decreased appetites. As they age, many older people prefer smaller portions. But they still need to eat regularly. Weight loss can be a sign of bad things to come. While the first concern raised by unintentional weight loss might be cancer, a variety of factors can contribute to decreased eating. Yes, some loss of appetite is related to disease. But it can just as easily be an innocent side effect of growing older.

Loss of Taste Sensation

Aging can cause a decrease in taste sensation, especially for sweet and salty flavors. Some medications and smoking can exacerbate this. As a result, older people may need to add more sugar or salt than is good for them, just to get the remembered taste. Add to that the bland food hospitals are notorious for serving and it is easy to see why elderly patients may find their hospital meals essentially tasteless. Even if their sense of taste is relatively unaffected, older people living in institutions may find the food choices unfamiliar or simply unappetizing. Obviously, both these factors can cause older people to eat less.

Preventing Choking: Pureed Diets Can Backfire

If nursing home staff or family members are concerned about aspiration (choking, not hope),[12] older patients may be put on special pureed diets. As you can probably imagine, these are not exactly Cordon Bleu cuisine. Institutions like nursing homes act out of a need for safety, but the trade-offs need to be considered. Institutionalized older people have few pleasures; food may be one of them. Many patients refuse pureed meals, and coaxing them into eating is a constant struggle. Preventing aspiration by starvation is a little bit like cutting off your nose to spite your face, and it's certainly not always in your loved one's best interest. Those who care for older people (in both senses of the word) need to carefully weigh the value of pureed diets.

Speech therapists do most of the swallowing assessments. They can often provide some useful advice about how to eat slowly and avoid distractions.

My mother had periodic episodes of choking, which were evaluated when she was in the nursing home and found to be related to aspiration. The nursing staff insisted that her liquids be thickened and her food pureed. We countered that what little remained of her quality of life would be severely compromised. (I urge anyone to try thickened tea before recommending it to someone.) But they were adamant. Even when we offered to sign waivers of liability, they responded that their license would be in jeopardy if she had an aspirational event.

Older People Should Be Allowed to Feed Themselves When Possible

Patients who can no longer feed themselves are also likely to eat less. It is frustrating to be fed, and many feeders are impatient or demean the older patient's very real needs. Feeding may be the fastest way to get

---

12. Aspiration implies literally inhaling food or liquid into your windpipe and causing choking. If the food is not exhaled by the choking and coughing, this can lead to pneumonia. Aspirating large chunks of food can block the windpipe and cause death.

older patients to eat, but speed shouldn't be the top priority. Wherever possible, older patients should be encouraged to feed themselves. Who cares if it takes a long time and makes a mess? So what if it takes more than an hour to finish a meal? Nursing aides who are expected to care for a complement of residents in a nursing home may feel great pressure to get them through meals as quickly as possible. They are hence likely to feed them and get the job done as quickly as possible, making mealtime a chore, not an event. Many institutions are reluctant to assign staff members to supervise, but that concern shouldn't trump concerns about forcing elderly patients to become overly dependent on others. One way many institutions reconcile the two concerns is by hiring feeding assistants whose job it is to oversee people eating, and, if truly necessary, to feed them.

How to Handle Food Shopping

For older people still living on their own, factors like having difficulty shopping for food and preparing meals can affect how much they eat. One solution is to arrange for home-delivered meals. Most communities have at least one meal delivery program (like Meals On Wheels). Some older people like this food, but it does not suit everyone's tastes. Prepared frozen food is easily available, so it is simple enough to fill a freezer with prepared meals that an older person will enjoy. Most of these can be heated in a microwave. Even older men who have hardly seen the inside of a kitchen can learn to use a microwave.

COMMUNICATE CHANGES TO THE DOCTOR

You may want to tell the medical professionals about issues with nutritional status, sleep, ability to perform activities of daily living, and emotional status. They will not always ask about these things. However, alerting them to such problems may lead to them prescribing more medication if something is out of whack, so tread lightly and be resourceful about finding non-drug-related solutions.

—DEB PAONE, CAREGIVING DAUGHTER

The Scale Does Not Lie

Like many problems with older people, there is a fine line between the kind of decrease in appetite you should worry about and the kind you should overlook. Be alert for signs of weight loss, like loose clothing. The best approach is to monitor the care recipient's weight. When changes occur, figure out why and respond appropriately.

When Loneliness Prevents Eating

Another common reason older people fail to eat is that they are alone. Preparing meals and eating them alone is difficult for some people. They are not interested in cooking simply for themselves. If this is the case, try to find a group dining experience. Many senior centers offer noon meals. Even better, have dinner together as often as possible. If you are going to visit, do it around a meal. Eat in or out, but eat together.

Impediments to Eating: Dental Problems, Fear of Money Shortage, and Depression

Dental problems, such as jaw pain or pain on chewing, or loose-fitting dentures, can change an older person's eating habits. Another obvious but often overlooked reason that older people eat less is a real or imagined lack of money. Older people may be unwilling to spend the money on food. If they will not buy it, you may have to.

Loss of appetite can also be a symptom of depression. This can be a cycle of despair. Isolation is associated with depression and with poor appetite. It can also be a sign of dementia. Confusion about how to prepare food may be hidden by simply not doing it.

Various Forms of Self-Neglect

Failing to eat properly may be a sign of self-neglect. But it is not the only one. Self-neglect can show itself through the way an older person fails to attend to any number of activities of daily living that were once simple routine. There are many reasons that older people often allow their personal appearances and their surroundings to become messy. Dementia can make people less aware of their environment and vision problems can complicate this. Dramatic changes in patterns of housekeeping, bathing, dressing, and other aspects of personal grooming should be carefully observed by caregivers, and responded to in appropriate ways.

Excessive Clutter

Outsiders are often shocked by the bric-a-brac cluttering the apartments of many older people. Children can be alarmed to find their formerly fastidious parents living in messy homes filled with jumbled collections. They see the piles of possessions as environmental hazards, and worry about falls. This concern is not entirely unjustified, but it is also important to appreciate that older people find their "messy" surroundings familiar and comfortable. Overly aggressive tidying that seriously alters their setups can be upsetting.

Bathing and Undressing

Bathing can be a problem for older people. Getting in and out of a tub can be painful and risky. Tubs are slippery and have high sides that present major obstacles to people with poor balance and weak muscles. Just pulling oneself up from lying in a bath is difficult for many older people. Pulling oneself up on a slippery surface is even harder. Adaptive devices like rails can be attached to the sides of tubs and safety bath mats are easy to get. (There are even specially built tubs you can walk into, but they are expensive and obviously require new plumbing.) Nonetheless, even with these adaptive devices, it is often much easier and safer to use showers, especially with a shower stool. It is not hard to adapt a shower to use a flexible hose. However, most older persons do not have separate showers. Instead, the shower is in the tub, and the same hazards apply.

Thus, older people may require assistance with bathing. This can be a very intrusive act. Perhaps second only to using the toilet, bathing is private. It requires nakedness. Depending on who the caregiver is, it can mean a lot of exposure and needs to be approached with sensitivity and respect.

Meeting Challenges for Independent Dressing

Dressing involves both physical and cognitive ability. Depending on our nature (and sense of style), a lot goes into choosing our wardrobe each day. Putting on clothes can be a problem-solving task that requires varying levels of dexterity (both physical and mental). I always marvel at how women can attach so many things behind their backs! For a person with arthritis or for someone recovering post-stroke, these tasks are major challenges. For a person with dementia, the choices of what to wear or how to put it on may be overwhelming.

Assistance with dressing comes in many forms. Persons with dementia may need cuing and reminding to get them to dress themselves. They may need help in selecting appropriate outfits. Persons with physical limitations may benefit from simpler fasteners like Velcro.

Ideally, older people should be encouraged to do as much for themselves as possible. A key factor in helping people is often time. It may take much longer for an older person to dress herself than to have it done for her. Another concern for some caregivers is appearance. How well can they tolerate shirts buttoned askew or mismatched outfits?

Simplifying Wardrobes

One solution is to simplify. All my life, I thought of my mother as a painstakingly chic dresser. As long as I could remember, she had a fastidious sense of clothes; each outfit was carefully planned. She passed this clothes sense on to my sister, who was then initially appalled when my mother needed to wear easily washable outfits because of her increasingly messy habits. As her dementia progressed and her eating became sloppier, my mother had to wear washable tracksuits made of fabrics that withstand the temperatures required by institutional laundries. But my sister learned to adapt, in part because my mother seemed quite happy in her new wardrobe. Ultimately, this compromise had many advantages. My mother could pretty much dress herself, and when she got dirty eating she could change her clothes several times a day, and everything was washable.

Inadequate Personal Grooming

People with dementia sometimes wear the same clothes every day, perhaps because it's easier. As a result they may end up wearing dirty clothes and the same underwear for days. And failing vision can cause the elderly to literally fail to see the dirt on themselves, their clothes, or their surroundings. Formerly dapper individuals may become unkempt and smelly. For children, this change can be pretty disorienting. Caregivers need to assess when to step in and when to give their loved one a little space.

Self-Neglect and Depression

Self-neglect can also be a symptom of depression. If other symptoms exist, like poor appetite, sleeping problems (too much or too little), and feeling sad, you might want to encourage your parent to seek treatment. It is important to watch for these warning signs. While some older people will admit to feeling blue when asked, others are reluctant to admit their feelings or believe those feelings are simply part of normal aging. (A full discussion of depression in the elderly, along with a checklist for assessing the warning signs of depression, can be found in Chapter Six.)

Keeping a Safe Home

Homes can be dangerous places, especially for older people with poor eyesight and balance problems. There is a great urge to sweep in and set things right. Simple home checklists, like Table 5.1, can help to identify things to look for. But do not expect changing things to be easy. Many older people like their clutter; it is what they consider part of home. Even

I resist my children coming in and "straightening things up." Here again, choose your battles carefully. Go after the really risky stuff and perhaps leave some of the neatness issues alone. For some older people strategic placement of furniture and other things may be major guides to navigation. Be careful what you change. One thing that older people often neglect is good lighting. Reduced vision can be helped by even stronger lighting than you may think necessary. Increasing wattage or using newer, more powerful bulbs may help. Sometimes you need more strategically placed lights. Automatic lights set to motion sensors can help. Grab bars that use suction are easy to install and move. Good-quality grab bars provide a lot of useful assistance with using the toilet and showering. Table 5.2 provides some ideas of things of consider to make an older person's house easier to negotiate.

Table 5.1: Home Safety Checklist

Windows and Doors	
1.	Are windows/doors easy to open and close?
2.	Are the locks sturdy and easy to operate?
3.	Are the doors wide enough for a walker or wheelchair?
4.	Are the door thresholds too high?
5.	Is there space to maneuver while opening or closing the doors?
6.	Does the front door have a view panel? Is it at a proper height for your loved one?
Floors	
1.	Is the surface safe and nonslip?
2.	Are there scatter rugs or doormats that may be dangerous?
3.	Are there changes in levels? If so, are they clearly marked?
Steps, Stairs, and Walkways	
1.	Are they in good repair?
2.	Do they have smooth, safe surfaces?

Table 5.1 (continued)

3.	Are there handrails on both sides of the stairway?
4.	Is there grasping space for both knuckles and fingers on the railings?
5.	Are the stair treads deep enough for your loved one's whole foot?
6.	Are there any hazardous open risers on the stairs?
7.	Would a ramp be feasible in any of these areas should the need arise?
	Appliances, Kitchen, and Bath
1.	Is the arrangement convenient and safe?
2.	Can the oven and refrigerator be opened easily?
3.	Are the stove controls easy to use? Are they clearly marked?
4.	Is the counter height/depth convenient for your loved one? Can he or she sit while working?
5.	Are the cabinet knobs easy to use?
6.	Are the faucets easy to use?
7.	Does your loved one have convenience items such as a garbage disposal? Trash compactor? Handheld shower head?
8.	Can your loved one get in and out of the tub or shower with ease?
9.	Does your loved one have a bath or shower seat?
10.	Are there grab bars where needed?
11.	Is the hot water heater regulated to prevent scalding?
	Storage
1.	Is the storage located conveniently?
2.	Is the storage adequate and usable?
3.	Can your loved one easily reach closet items?
4.	Has your loved one maximized storage space with innovative products?

Table 5.1 (continued)

	Electrical Outlets, Switches, and Alarms
1.	Are the outlets/switches easy to turn off and on?
2.	Are the outlets properly grounded to prevent electrical shock?
3.	Are the extension cords in good condition? Are they needed?
4.	Does your loved one have smoke detectors in all the necessary areas?
5.	Does your loved one have an alarm system?
6.	Is the telephone readily available for emergencies?
7.	Is the telephone equipped for hearing enhancement, if necessary?
8.	Can your loved one hear the doorbell in every part of the house?

Table 5.2: Simple Things to Make a Home Safer

1.	Adjustable closet rods.
2.	A night-light in the bedroom.
3.	Area rugs removed.
4.	Handrails on both sides of staircases and outside steps.
5.	Brighter staircase lighting.
6.	Large rocker light switches that turn on and off with a push.
7.	Electric outlets twenty-seven inches from the floor.
8.	Peephole or view panel in the front door.
9.	Walk-in shower with grab bars and portable or adjustable shower seat.
10.	Handheld adjustable shower head.
11.	Nonskid surface for bathtub and shower floor.
12.	Grab bars by the toilet and tub.
13.	Tilting or full-length mirror in the bathroom.
14.	Bathroom telephone that is reachable should your loved one fall.

Table 5.2 (continued)

15.	Adjustable countertops or lower counter for work space in the kitchen.
16.	Kitchen countertops with rounded edges.
17.	Sliding shelves in cupboards; lazy Susan in the corner cabinet.
18.	First-floor bedroom and bath to allow living entirely on one level, if necessary.

Exercise and Quality of Life

Exercise is good for people. It may not only make people fit (or at least fitter), it can be a good social activity. Exercise has been shown to postpone disability and improve one's sense of health. Even nursing home residents have been seen to benefit from mild exercise. Building regimens that encourage moderate regular exercise of the upper and lower body is a good idea. The key concepts are **moderate** and **regular**. Ideally such exercise can be done in a group for several reasons. (1) It is more likely to be done if done with others. (2) It encourages socialization. Walking is good exercise. For people who live in places with severe winters, mall walking can work well. Most senior centers and Y's have senior adult exercise programs. Not all older people will take to this idea. Some may need encouragement; you may even need to go with them in the beginning.

In the Bedroom: Sex and the Elderly

Most adults do not like to imagine their parents having sex. Maybe they harbor some idea about divine creation to explain their own existence. In popular mythology sex among older people is treated as a joke. But that does not mean older people stop getting it on. Alex Comfort, a well known gerontologist, tried to break the taboo around later-life sex by publishing a matter-of-fact book on the subject, *A Good Age*, (Crown Publishers, 1976). He had limited success, however. His book did more to titillate than to make the topic less illicit.

Despite the jokes, many older people, including nursing home residents, pursue sexual activity. Many institutions view such interest as disruptive, inappropriate, and even immoral. The staff will often go to great lengths to prohibit and even punish any kind of sexual activity. Talk about diminishing the quality of life!

Coming to Terms with Sexuality in Older Persons

Children and especially caregivers must be prepared to deal with the awkward idea that their parents still want to have sex. If family members are uncomfortable with the idea that their elderly loved ones might want to make some whoopee, this will just reinforce institutions' preexisting tendencies to ban sex. Dementia can fuel the flames burning around this already sensitive subject. Dementia can lower inhibitions, so patients may behave in unorthodox ways. Public masturbation, fondling, and other expressions of affection may occur. The skill and tact with which these are managed will impact an older person's quality of life. Signals from family members can shape the institution's response. If family members treat this behavior as normal, which it is, institutions will follow suit. However, if family members act embarrassed, patients may be discouraged and even shamed.

Sex and Drugs

The relationship between sex and drugs changes with age. For teenagers one worries that drugs lead to sex. Older persons may need drugs to help them have sex. Male impotence is a major contributor to decreasing sexual activity in older people. Fortunately for older men and women everywhere, drugs like Viagra and Cialis are now widely available. But these drugs do have risks. It might be time to reverse that old talk about the birds and the bees.

Chapter Five—Points to Ponder

Giving up driving is not easy. The loss of independence that accompanies retiring one's driver's license is a life-changing event. It may take a lot of convincing. Be persistent. Get help from influential sources.

Self-neglect can be serious. Be observant for signs of self-neglect.

Pleasure in eating matters. Weigh the risks of aspiration against the pleasures of eating.

Home safety requires attention. Make simple environmental changes to make an older person's home safer.

Six

Common Ailments
and Treatments

Aging entails certain physical changes; many are inevitable. But the inevitability of the changes is no reason not to respond to and treat the discomforts and ailments aging can cause. Effort should be made to make aging a more pleasant and better tolerated experience. Caregivers should not assume that a complaint is just an inevitable discomfort of growing old. Any complaints could signal a serious health problem or an acute condition requiring specific treatment. Some complaints can be alleviated altogether with appropriate care.

Chronic disease is a central part of frailty. Managing chronic disease well can minimize that frailty and hopefully prevent catastrophes that lead to hospitalizations and the attendant risks. Chronic disease is big business. It accounts for 80 percent of health care spending (almost 95 percent for older people). No wonder lots of people are working on ways to treat it.

Even as you are reading this, researchers are developing new drugs and interventions tailored to elderly patients. For example, new guidelines have been developed around screening for colorectal cancer and diabetes among elderly men and women. Prevention of injuries or health risk based on heredity and genes is another hot area for research. Certain drugs can help prevent cancer. Changes in diet and lifestyle help control or treat high blood pressure. A carefully planned exercise program and a well-balanced home-care approach can bring new order into the life of elderly people and reduce hospital admissions. Creative new ways of delaying the onset of disease and disability are reducing morbidity and mortality among the elderly. As a caregiver for an older person, you need to know how to respond to some of the most common ailments. You need to know when you can administer a remedy yourself and when a medical examination is more advisable.

Disease Presentation

Diseases often present differently in older people. The signs and symptoms are more subtle. Most symptoms of a disease reflect your body's responses to the stresses the disease is inflicting on you. One of the hallmarks of aging is a reduced capacity to respond to stress. Baseline physiological values, like heart rate and white blood cell counts, are the same in older people and younger. However, when a problem arises, the older person may not respond the same way.

Symptoms of the same disease look different for a thirty-year-old and for a seventy-year-old. Because many symptoms are not the manifestations of the disease per se but rather the body's response to the insult and the failure to respond to stress is a hallmark of aging, it follows that such symptoms and signs will be muted. A fever is the body's response to toxic substances, and increase in white blood cells is a response to infection. But when faced with either of these problems, an older body is less likely to develop a fever or mount a white blood cell increase. This makes it harder for a doctor to find the root cause of an older person's sickness, especially if she fails to appreciate that diseases manifest themselves differently in older patients.

The problem of diagnosing new conditions in older persons is complicated by the existence of multiple underlying conditions. Whereas a new problem in a younger person may be compared to a mountain on a plain, such problems in an older person are like noting the emergence of a new alp.

The I's of Geriatrics

Because diseases can present in atypical ways, interpreting a symptom or behavior in an older person can be hazardous. The same symptom can reflect many different underlying problems. We talk about the "I's of geriatrics," a series of conditions whose names start with the letter *i*, listed below.

Immobility	Instability
Intellectual impairment	Insomnia
Incontinence	Inanition (poor appetite)
Impairment of hearing or vision	Isolation (depression)
Infection	Impecunity
Impotence	Immune deficiency
Iatrogenesis (result of treatment)	

Each can be the manifestation of many disparate problems. For example, older persons may be immobile because they have severe arthritis that makes walking difficult. But they may also not walk much because they get short of breath from congestive heart failure. Some problems are due to diseases; others are exacerbated (or even created) by the environment in which a person lives. People with severe congestive heart failure may be rendered unable to leave the house if they live up two flights of stairs and have no elevator.

A few bear special mention. "Iatrogenesis" refers to problems created by treatment. Treating older patients constantly requires trading potential gain for harm. The window that separates the likelihood of positive versus negative effects narrows with age. Clinicians (and by extension families) must always keep in mind that every treatment poses a risk, but neither can they become paralyzed by fear to treat.

Impotence has two connotations here. Earlier we discussed the role of sex in the lives of older people. Impotence is often iatrogenic, secondary to drugs; but it can be iatrogenic in another sense as well. Older people can be made to feel powerless if all decisions and control are removed from their grasp. It is is all too easy to fall into this trap, acting in their stead because it is easier and faster.

Vision and Hearing

It is normal for our vision to change as we age. The lens of the eye loses its plasticity with age and cannot change shape to accommodate to near and far vision as easily as it once could. At some point, most people will need glasses to see things up close, far away, or both. But some diseases cause more serious visual impairment. Vision loss can be an ongoing side effect of chronic diseases like diabetes. Vision loss is also commonly caused by three other diseases: glaucoma, macular degeneration, and cataracts. Glaucoma attacks peripheral vision, macular degeneration destroys central vision, and cataracts blur everything. In effect, these three diseases affect vision from all sides.

Cataracts

Cataracts are imperfections in the lens of the eye. They impair the transmission of light. A frequent symptom is trouble with night vision, especially halos around lights. Cataracts may also cause blurry vision, faded color perception, and double vision. Over time, they cause substantial vision loss. In the past, it was necessary to wait until a cataract was "ripe"—so advanced that the patient was nearly blind—before cataract surgery could be performed. However, medical advances have made the surgery much safer and more convenient. It is now possible for cataract sufferers to essentially choose for themselves when they would like to have their cataracts removed. The procedure can be done as same-day surgery. As with all serious care, take the time to check out the surgeon. Not only should she be a boarded ophthalmologist, cataract replacement should be a subspecialty. This is an area where volume matters. Ask to see data on her outcomes, including complication rates.

Glaucoma

Glaucoma affects the fluids behind the lens of the eye. It increases the pressure within the eye, which in turn impairs peripheral vision. So, a smaller field of vision is a solid indicator of glaucoma. Glaucoma has two forms—acute and chronic; the latter is much more common, but the former is a medical emergency. Drugs that control the production and excretion of fluid, which changes the pressure within the eye, can be used to treat chronic glaucoma. These drugs interact with a number of medications and other diseases, especially chronic lung disease. Discuss these medications in the context of everything the patient is taking. Acute glaucoma, however, may require surgery.

Macular Degeneration

Loss of function in the macula is called age-related macular degeneration, or AMD. The macula is part of the retina, located in the back part of the eye. It produces the most detailed vision. So AMD results in a loss of central vision. Early symptoms include straight lines appearing wavy or crooked. AMD occurs in two forms—wet and dry. There is no treatment for the more common dry variety, but there are some promising treatments for the wet form.

Hearing Loss

An elderly gentleman named Bob walks into a doctor's office. After becoming virtually deaf, he finally invested in a hearing aid, one of the virtually invisible ones. "Well, Bob, how do you like your new hearing aid?" asks his doctor.

"I like it great. I've heard sounds in the last few weeks that I didn't know existed."

"Well, how does your family like your hearing aid?"

"Oh, nobody in my family knows I have it yet. Am I having a great time! I've changed my will three times in the last two months."

Joking aside, loss of hearing and old age often go hand in hand. There are two basic types of hearing loss: conduction problems and nerve damage. Conduction problems are more common and fortunately are easier to treat. Conduction refers to the process by which the sound waves enter the ear and are conveyed to the inner ear, where they are transformed in nerve impulses. Blockages of the ear canal (e.g., wax buildup) or fusion of the tiny bones that transmit the sound can affect hearing. Essentially, conduction loss impedes older people from distinguishing between the sound of someone speaking to them and the sound of background noise. One of the hallmarks of conduction deafness is the inability to hear well in a crowd.

Conduction deafness can be treated with amplification hearing aids. Amplification works in two ways: first, overall volume is increased, and second, sound is conducted through the bone. This offsets the faults in the traditional conduction pathways.

New and Improved Hearing Aids

We have come a long way from the days when a hearing aid was a trumpet you held up to your ear for people to shout into. One of the most important advances has been how hearing tests are conducted. Typical hearing tests check for the ability to hear different frequencies and amplitudes, but the actual process of hearing is much more complex. Hearing requires the brain to transform noises into meaningful messages. Newer tests account for this step, and focus on hearing words rather than just tones. Hearing aids have been seriously upgraded as well. Early hearing aids were bulky and uncomfortable. They simply made everything louder. Today hearing aids are technological marvels. "Invisible" hearing aids (like Bob's) are not just discreet, they are also elaborately constructed to allow selective filtering for different frequencies. You can adjust them to compensate for the specific frequencies where you have lost hearing. Typically the higher frequencies are lost first. This is one reason why someone with hearing impairment might have more difficulty hearing a woman's voice than a man's. Obviously, hearing aids cannot solve all hearing problems. But they can make a big difference.

Overcoming Hearing Aid Resistance

Of course hearing aids help hearing only if they are worn. Unfortunately, many older people do not want to use hearing aids. Vanity is part of the problem. When many elderly people picture hearing aids, the image that comes to mind is the old box with a wire to your ear. Another stumbling block is that many older people are not willing to spend the time learning how to properly use their hearing aids. Some older people complain that new hearing aids emit an unpleasant whining noise. However, proper adjustment can solve this problem. And ironically, hearing aid miniaturization has created new problems. People with tremors or arthritis may have trouble inserting the device into their ear. Likewise, for people with vision problems, changing the tiny batteries, which need frequent replacement, can be tricky. In the face of these obstacles, many old people grow frustrated and toss the vexing hearing aids into a drawer alongside their dentures and eyeglasses. This makes it easy for caregivers to ignore the issue. Do not do this. It may take a lot of support and coaxing from caregivers to help older people master hearing aids, but it is worth it. Once older people get the use of the hearing aid down pat, their ability to attend to day-to-day activities, as well as the quality of their social interactions, can be dramatically improved.

Osteoporosis

Old bones become brittle and thin. Many older people suffer from osteoporosis, basically a loss of bone density. Thin, white women with a family history of slender bones are at the greatest risk for osteoporosis. Fortunately, osteoporosis can be treated. At a minimum, all older people, especially older women, should take calcium and vitamin D supplements and exercise regularly.[13] There is a specific test for osteoporosis. The density of your bones can be measured with no pain or inconvenience. The

---

13. Osteoporosis affects men, too.

test is done with a dual photon emission screen. The test works like an X-ray, except that it uses a somewhat different type of machine and very little radiation. The results are reported as T scores, which reflect how a person's score compares to a large panel of healthy people of the same age and sex. A score substantially different from the comparison group, usually a T score of −2.5 or less, indicates a need for treatment. A bone fracture can also indicate osteoporosis, although not all fractures are triggered by weak bones. There is a program under way to start all patients with hip fractures on treatment for osteoporosis.

Osteoporosis Treatment

People who suffer from osteoporosis should be on bisphosphonate medications like Fosamax. However, not everyone with a low T score needs these medications. They are best used by those with substantially low scores (below −2.5). These medications alter bone metabolism to slow bone loss. Because these medications can cause stomach upset or heartburn, you must sit upright for thirty to sixty minutes afterward to prevent gastric reflux. And conveniently enough, some of these medications need to be taken only once a month. One variation must be taken (actually injected) only once a year. However, even if they are taking the new bisphosphonate drugs to treat their osteoporosis, many older people's bones remain weak, meaning that they have a high risk of breaking a hip.

Hip Fracture

It is easier to break your hip if your bones are thin. In some cases, a fall may lead to a broken bone. But in other cases, just the reverse occurs and a break leads to a fall. Imagine an older woman stepping off a curb to cross the street. The impact of stepping down causes her hip to fracture, and that fracture causes her to fall to the ground.

Breaking a hip can have serious health consequences. Often, a hip fracture marks the beginning of the end. Sometimes it marks a gradual loss of independence, sometimes it marks a rapid decline. Either way, hip fracture patients have high mortality rates. At least a third of all hip fracture patients will die within a year. However, it is not clear whether this frightening death rate is caused by the hip fractures per se, or whether it reflects the fact that older people who fall and fracture their hips are often very frail. It is hard to separate the underlying risks of frailty from the added dangers created by the fracture, but the danger remains.

Hip Fracture Treatment

One reason hip fractures have such damaging consequences is that they need to be repaired surgically. There are several different approaches, ranging from putting in a pin (a fairly large piece of metal that holds the broken bone together), to using external fixation (a system of plates and screws that provides support while the fracture heals), to replacing the hip joint. You should talk to an orthopedic surgeon about the pros and cons of each approach. One important factor is recovery time. The sooner the older person can begin walking again, the better. It is important to consult very soon after a hip fracture with a physical therapist to design and implement a recovery program. Ideally this rehabilitation starts while the patient is still in the hospital. Overly cautious management can make it very difficult for an older patient to fully recover from a hip fracture. Hip fracture patients are often placed on bed rest afterward. This restriction can lead to further deconditioning and disability. A worst-case scenario is that a hip fracture patient is catheterized because getting to the bathroom is a problem. Catheterization can spawn a whole host of problems (see the section on iatrogenic disease, page 202).

Encouraging Hip Fracture Recovery

Recovering from a hip fracture takes time, effort, and determination from older patients and caregivers. Not every elderly person is up to the task, but in almost every case, you should encourage the care recipient to try. A hip fracture can be the straw that breaks the camel's back. Sometimes a frail older person will simply be unwilling to face further deterioration. If they are truly ready for the end, it can be a mistake to push them through the grueling process of recovery. But it's also a mistake to give up on someone—or allow them to give up on themselves—before they have given rehabilitation a good shot. Some of the consequences of a hip fracture are mental, not physical. People who have fallen and injured themselves can be fearful about the possibility of falling again. They might try to protect themselves by not walking. Just like an unreasonably long period of bed rest, this fear can be an impediment to recovery.

Preventing Hip Fracture

Breaking a hip opens up a Pandora's box full of troubles; so obviously it is preferable to avoid falls and fractures. However, efforts to prevent falls are difficult and there's no way to guarantee they'll work. Various exercises have been tried, but the benefits are mixed. Balance training is probably the most effective, but the size of the benefit is still modest. Drugs that create unsteadiness (drugs to improve mood and sedatives, for example) should be avoided whenever possible. Another prevention strategy is to get older people to wear specially designed hip protectors. These protectors are designed to prevent a fracture if an older person does fall. But it is hard to convince older people to wear these cumbersome protectors, and research shows that they have only a limited ability to prevent fractures.

Common sense can tell you that creating a safer environment will help prevent falls. Eliminate things like loose rugs and wires, install grab bars in bathrooms, and improve lighting. Avoid slippery surfaces, like wet leaves and icy paths. And rule out the possibility of an older person tripping over her own feet by purchasing sensible footwear that fits well and provides support. Resources providing more ideas about ways to make a home safer can be found in the appendix.

UNCLE JOE AT AGE ONE HUNDRED

Uncle Joe—actually he was my dad's uncle, so my great-uncle—lived alone until he was one hundred years old. He farmed on the Iowa/Minnesota border until his son took over the farm. Uncle Joe had the broadest hands that I have ever seen. Even at one hundred years of age, Uncle Joe made you wince when he shook your hand. Uncle Joe was as Catholic as they come. In fact, everyone he knew was identified by the religion that they practiced. For instance, Josephine, the Baptist, was very kind to him after he could no longer drive. He grew flowers in her yard and in the yard of the church across the street from his home. Uncle Joe knew what each of his children, grandchildren, and great-grandchildren were doing and where they lived. One of the local women delivered a pie to his home every Saturday. This way, he had a piece of pie every day. Uncle Joe had had multiple medical problems including prostate cancer. He had each of his hips replaced, with a total hip two times. When he was one hundred, one of the hip sockets fractured and, because of his age, the doctors would not replace the hip a third time. Uncle Joe could only take a step or two, so went to live at a nursing home. He said, "It's not so bad once you get the staff trained." It was always a treat to visit Uncle Joe because he continued to be very interested in others and in life.

—JOANN HOWITZ, CAREGIVER AND PHYSICAL THERAPIST

DON'T OVERLIMIT MOBILITY

In the nursing home where I worked as a physical therapist, there was a resident named John who was able to walk the long halls in the nursing home with his cane. Thanksgiving came and his family came to visit me to request a wheelchair to take him home for Thanksgiving. I explained to John's daughter that John was able to go up and down stairs and that he could walk the distances needed to go home. The daughter replied, "Oh, don't say that. My mother is in a wheelchair and it is so cute to see the two of them in wheelchairs!" I am still surprised that my rehab heart survived that one!

—JOANN HOWITZ, CAREGIVER AND PHYSICAL THERAPIST

Overprotection and Fall Phobia

At the other extreme, excessive fall phobia (among either older persons or those caring for them) can be disastrous, too. Some nursing homes, for example, are so afraid of having residents fall that they restrict their movement. Confining an older person unnecessarily to a wheelchair (or even worse, an immovable chair) is a very high price to pay. One of the frequent dilemmas in caring for frail older people is determining how much risk they can and should take. Taking risks is part of life. Living a risk-free life can be very sterile and limiting. The trick is to understand the risks and make informed choices.

Don't Tie Up Older People

Physical restraints are an inappropriate prevention strategy. Physical restraints are usually used to prevent an older person from getting out of bed, or in some cases, prevent them from pulling out tubes or IVs. Too often, frail older people are tied up or tied down. It can be an instinctive response to protect an older person by restraining them, but it's also the wrong response. Unfortunately, many misguided family members push for the use of restraints. Keeping older people tied in chairs, or in bed, is not only a poor way to treat another human being, it's a poor way to prevent falls. Restraints can cause more falls than they prevent. Fortunately, restraints are falling out of favor. There is growing agreement among professionals that very strong justification is required for any use of restraints. Nevertheless, many practitioners still believe that restraints are an important safety measure. This is simply not true. Restraints are not only demeaning, they are dangerous. This prohibition applies to more subtle restraints as well, such as geri-chairs, which keep people confined.

Joint Replacement

Theoretically, it is possible to replace almost all of the two-hundred-plus joints in the human body. These days, joint replacement surgery is becoming

Joint Replacement Tips

Here is some straight talk and practical advice from people who have had joint replacement surgeries:

- Find the right surgeon. Look for one with excellent credentials and a strong record of positive outcomes as well as a positive attitude.
- Be sure that nails, especially toenails, are trimmed short and perfect before surgery. It will be weeks before to the patient can get to them on her own again!
- Arrange round-the-clock caregiving for at least three weeks.
- Remember to request prescribed pain pills on time (that is, before pain kicks in) and be sure to cut back and cut off pill use as soon as possible.
- Be prepared to deal with constipation as a result of taking pain pills.
- Insist on aggressive physical therapy, beginning the day of surgery.
- Arrange that the car for the trip home from the hospital is an SUV. These cars allow the patient easiest access. The patient should sit on a plastic bag facing straight out the door and then turn forward (or have someone position the patient by lifting from under both knees simultaneously) to reduce friction between clothing and the car seat cover.
- Have the following "assistive devices" at home and have the older person become comfortable with them before surgery takes place. Every single one is essential!

    - Raised toilet seat and toilet frame (these have handles to push up on).

    - Wheelchair with detachable feet. Test-drive the wheelchair before surgery to be sure it can get the patient into the bathroom from the bed, turn, and back to bed on his own.

    - Shower bench and portable showerhead.

    - Ice, from a machine if possible, or large ice bags at minimum, to minimize swelling. The effect is enhanced when you dampen (not soak) a washcloth or pillowcase and put it between the ice pack and your surgery site.

    - Cart to move the ice machine from kitchen to bedroom and large disposable pads (from grocery or drugstore) to place under your legs and protect your floors while cooling the surgery site.

If you keep this advice in mind, you can avoid or eliminate many of the common problems resulting from joint replacement surgery.

ever more common and less intrusive. The most common joints to be replaced are hips and knees. A hip replacement may mean replacing only the head of the femur (aka your thighbone) or the whole kit and caboodle may be replaced, the femur head and acetabulum (aka the ball and socket). Neither hip nor knee replacements will last forever. Adjustments (reoperations) are usually needed within ten to fifteen years. Newer replacement joints can last longer, however, especially for older people with less active lifestyles. Recovery from hip replacements is usually fairly easy, whereas recovery from a knee replacement requires more aggressive rehabilitation.

High Blood Pressure

Blood pressure is higher as people age. For a long time doctors argued about whether this was simply a normal component of the aging process or a pathological change. Many geriatricians felt that because anti-hypertensive drugs had serious side effects, it might be safer not to treat elevated blood pressure aggressively. The tide of opinion has changed dramatically. Hypertension is recognized as a major risk factor for heart disease and stroke. Diabetics are at special risk. Active efforts are aimed at keeping blood pressure within normal limits (a systolic pressure less than 120 mm Hg and a diastolic pressure no more than 80. (Blood pressure is typically reported as systolic/diastolic.) Some would urge even more stringent goals. Specific treatment regimens have been developed, usually based on some form of "stepped care" in which one starts with relatively innocuous drugs and adds more potent treatments only when the simple approaches do not work. Hypertension is a lifetime diagnosis. Treatment does not make it better; it simply controls it. The medication has to be taken regularly and essentially forever.

Gastroesophageal Reflux Disease (GERD)

Basically, GERD is a kind of heartburn. Highly acidic stomach contents are partially regurgitated into the esophagus, the tube that connects your mouth to your stomach. This damages the lining of the esophagus. Typical symptoms of GERD include indigestion, a chronic cough, upset stomach, and pain. GERD is treated with antacids, H_2 blockers (like Pepcid or Zantac), or proton pump inhibitors (like Nexium and Prilosec), and with behavioral and dietary changes. There is no one cause of GERD. Making a diagnosis can lead to better treatment, but it is often impossible to determine what is the actual cause. Overcoming GERD can require some lifestyle changes. Simple steps like raising the head of the bed by thirty degrees, refraining from eating for half an hour before bedtime, and avoiding greasy foods, caffeinated or alcoholic beverages, or any other foods that seem to exacerbate the problem can help significantly.

Urinary Incontinence

Urinary incontinence is a frequent problem for older people. Urinary incontinence simply means the leakage of urine. Studies show that more than 50 percent of women and about 20 percent of men over age sixty-five suffer from some degree of incontinence. The figure is even higher for nursing home residents—up to 75 percent of nursing home patients who remain in the home longer than ninety days suffer from incontinence. Incontinence varies in intensity from an urgent and frequent need to pee to the actual leakage of varying amounts of urine. This leakage might be a little release with a cough, laugh, or sneeze, or a complete emptying of the bladder. Urinary incontinence is classified into various types.

Stress Incontinence

Stress incontinence is basically a failure of the mechanisms that keep urine in the bladder. This can be caused by many things. One of the most common causes is weak pelvic muscles, which in turn are often the result of pregnancies. Sphincter problems, a frequent side effect of prostate surgery, are another top cause of stress incontinence. With stress incontinence, urinary leakage occurs when abdominal pressure increases. This is why a sneeze or cough often triggers leakage.

Overflow Incontinence

A second form of incontinence is overflow incontinence. Overflow incontinence is caused by the failure of the bladder to empty completely. This builds up a reservoir of unpassed urine. Overflow incontinence is usually due to a sphincter that can't adequately relax when a person is urinating, or to the failure of the bladder muscle to function in a coordinated way. It can also be caused by an obstruction, such as an enlarged prostate. Over time, the bladder will become distended. This makes proper emptying even more challenging.

Gotta Go, Gotta Go, Gotta Go!

Urgency incontinence is a slightly different form of overflow incontinence. People who suffer from urgency incontinence constantly feel like they need to pee, right now. Urgency incontinence may indicate an acute bladder infection or another local irritation, or may simply be what is termed an overactive bladder. Medications are available to help treat this problem.

How to Deal with Urinary Incontinence

Unfortunately, except for problems caused by urinary tract infections, urinary incontinence can rarely be cured. Most of the time, urinary incontinence just has to be managed. Some physicians are enthusiastic about surgical solutions such as pelvic floor suspension procedures for women and prostheses that typically clamp the urethra for men. Most of these procedures don't work as well as promised, and any benefits may come with unintended consequences. Be sure you have the full picture before agreeing to surgery. What is its overall record of success? What are the potential side effects? What is this surgeon's record? There are also drugs are available, both to stimulate bladder contraction and to enhance sphincter function. Once again, these drugs work moderately well at best, and can have severe side effects. For stress incontinence in women, special exercises called Kegels have proved very effective. These exercises strengthen the pelvic floor muscles, and with continued practice, substantial success has been seen. For urgency incontinence, behavior training—euphemistically called "mind over bladder"—might provide some relief. The most direct treatment (really management) for ongoing incontinence is timed toileting. This is simply the practice of encouraging a person to use the toilet on a regular schedule. This will not eliminate the incontinence. But if a person follows a set a schedule of regular bathroom visits, usually every couple of hours, it can prevent accidents.

Remember the I's of geriatrics. Some incontinence is situational. An old person who has trouble getting out of bed or who cannot walk easily may have a urinary accident simply because she cannot get to the toilet fast enough. This problem can be solved in several ways if you get to the root of the problem. Timed toileting is one answer. Another may be a bedside commode.

Adult Diapers

The very concept of an adult diaper is offensive to many people. In response to that, ambiguous euphemisms like "adult pads" and "urinary incontinence pads" are frequently substituted for the distasteful "d-word." Most older people find the idea of wearing a diaper or a special absorbent undergarment demeaning and infantilizing. The companies that manufacture adult diapers have actively campaigned against this stereotype. They claim that their products can liberate people with incontinence and allow them to lead more normal lives. In this case, the advertisements are true. On the downside, disposable adult diapers/underpants/panty liners are relatively expensive, and pose the same environmental concerns as infant diapers. Pads that can be worn inside the underwear are also available for sufferers of light leakage, usually from stress incontinence. Many people might not want to admit it, but adult diapers are widely used. If asked, most people who suffer from incontinence will reveal a variety of creative coping mechanisms for preventing urine from appearing on their clothes. If it helps, think of wearing diapers as part of a backup plan for your loved one, but it should not be the first line of defense. The worst thing that can happen is to have caregivers encourage older persons to urinate in their pants because they are wearing diapers.

What Not to Do for Incontinence

Controlling incontinence is important. Incontinence can greatly restrict social activity and hence quality of life. Not only is incontinence socially embarrassing and uncomfortable, persistent wetness can lead to skin breakdown and infection.

A nursing home resident can find it challenging to get staff to promptly answer a call bell and assist them to and from the toilet. Nursing home staff may complain about residents wanting to go to the toilet too often. Even after pressing the call bell, many older residents are made to wait for extended periods of time. Some get so frustrated and desperate that, despite warnings, they try to get to the bathroom on their own. This sad state of affairs can readily lead to a whole chain of mishaps ending in a hip fracture. Nursing home residents should not be put into situations where they must risk a fall or worse in order to use the toilet. Unfortunately, in many nursing homes, that is the way it is. It is not uncommon for nursing home staff to say to a resident, "Don't worry about getting to the toilet. You've got a diaper on—just go ahead and go in it!" This approach is not only infantilizing, it also opens the residents up to greater risk of skin breakdown—decubitus ulcers or "bedsores."

Perhaps the worst way to address incontinence is to insert a catheter into the bladder. This practice frequently leads to urinary tract infections, and with extended use, it practically ensures that the catheterized patient will never again be able to urinate normally.

Incontinence and Dementia

Sometimes people become incontinent for reasons not related to sphincter function or muscle control. Older people who suffer from advanced dementia may lose their inhibitions, including their sense of decorum about how to manage their bodily functions. They may urinate and even defecate in inappropriate locations. Clearly, this behavior can be very distressing for their caregivers. And not surprisingly, it regularly leads to institutional care. However, if the person with dementia is helped to use the toilet on a regular basis, institutional care can be avoided for longer. And that is always a good thing.

Fecal Incontinence

Fecal incontinence is less common than urinary incontinence, and it almost always occurs in conjunction with urinary incontinence. Fecal incontinence can come from two sources. The physical cause is basically the failure of the rectal sphincter. Depending on the extent of the failure, you can leak gas, liquid, or solid stool. Surgical repair can work in some cases, but there are no readily available devices or behavioral therapies to manage this form of incontinence.

Fecal incontinence can also be a sign of fecal impaction. In these cases, hardened stool blocks the rectum until some liquid leaks around the clog. Patients on bed rest are especially prone to fecal impaction. Older persons who are not having regular bowel movements, especially those who are very frail and unable to communicate, should be checked regularly for fecal impaction. Opiate medications are known to cause constipation. So if your loved one is taking these medications to manage pain, there may be a need for a daily pro-motility agent, such as sorbitol. However, stool softeners should be used only if absolutely necessary. Laxatives can be habit forming. After a while, they not only lose their effectiveness, they can actually cause digestive problems. A safer way to reduce the risk of suffering from fecal impaction is to be sure your loved one eats a diet rich in fiber and liquids.

The other cause of fecal incompetence is the failure to inhibit behavior. As noted above, persons suffering from dementia may become incontinent because they no longer adhere to bodily signs or simply lose their inhibitions about what is deemed proper behavior. This sort of incontinence is very hard to treat. Some efforts to use a variation of timed toileting may help along with dietary manipulation, but fecal incontinence among persons with dementia usually leads to institutionalization because caregivers simply cannot cope with it.

Diarrhea

Ironically, as you now know, fecal impaction can also cause fecal incontinence, a type of diarrhea. However, other types of diarrhea can be even more problematic. Diarrhea can be caused by excessive use of laxatives, a change in diet, or active use of antibiotics that kill the gut flora. In rare cases, it may be caused by a gastrointestinal (GI) infection. Diarrhea is not only annoying, it is dangerous. Older people with diarrhea can lose a great deal of fluid quickly. Older people compensate poorly for losses in fluids and electrolytes. Prolonged diarrhea can cause dehydration and electrolyte imbalance, serious problems for older people. Signs of weakness and confusion should be taken seriously.

Electrolyte Imbalance

Diarrhea is just one cause of electrolyte imbalance. Sustained diarrhea causes loss of important electrolytes, and in turn the body's pH balance (the measure of how much acid is in the blood) falls. The human body needs to maintain a steady level of electrolyte balance. Electrolyte balance is determined both by the body's pH and by the level of minerals in the bloodstream. A person's pH level measures acidity, and a low pH signifies more acid. In simple terms, our pH is determined by how much carbon dioxide we retain and by our digestive fluids. Our stomachs contain acids that are neutralized by lower portions of our digestive tract. This is why diarrhea causes your pH balance to drop. Conversely, if a person vomits a great deal, acid is lost (largely hydrochloric acid) and the body's pH rises.

Most people's bodies have automatic mechanisms to restore pH balance, but many older people's bodies lose the ability to respond quickly to stress. This makes them more susceptible to electrolyte imbalances. Electrolytes include basic chemicals like sodium, potassium, and chlorine. Electrolyte imbalances can affect mental status as well as physical status, causing weakness and confusion. If electrolyte levels are too low, intravenous fluids are needed to replace the lost electrolytes. And if electrolyte levels are too high, they will need to be diluted.

Dehydration

As people age, everything requires more effort. Older people burn a lot of energy just getting through the day. This means lower energy reserves, and a decreased ability to respond to stress, like dehydration. Dehydration affects electrolyte balance. In effect, the electrolytes are diluted by body fluids. If too much water is lost, the levels of the electrolytes rise. As the high death rates among older persons in heat waves show, dehydration can kill. A downward spiral can take over very quickly. Be extra cautious in hot weather. Even if the older person's temperature is not spiking, make sure your care recipient is consuming enough fluids. If an older person is feeling ill, he or she may not want to eat or drink much. They may lose fluids even faster if they have a fever. Diarrhea and vomiting cause loss of both fluids and electrolytes. An older person already perched on a narrow ledge of metabolic balance can quickly and quietly fall off.

Dehydration is subtle and thus frequently overlooked. It may look like many other things. It is amazing how a frail older person who seems on the point of death can be revived with a liter or so of fluid. A dehydrated older person may appear confused. An emergency room visit is a common response to acute confusion in an older person. Oftentimes, after the mess and stress of an emergency room visit, it turns out all that was required was some intravenous fluids.

Constipation

Constipation, the exact opposite of diarrhea, is one of the most common and annoying problems affecting older people. It can be exacerbated by inactivity, eating the wrong foods, not drinking enough fluids, and by some medications.

Unlike irritable bowel syndrome (IBS), constipation does not cause abdominal pain or straining at defecation. Constipation is just one of the many problems that crop up as we get older, but sometimes it is a symptom of a more serious problem, like colon cancer. If it is accompanied by a weight loss of ten pounds or more, an abdominal mass, or evidence of GI bleeding, it should be investigated.

The usual treatment for constipation begins with increasing fiber in the diet and increasing fluid intake. Eating more bran, fruits, and vegetables and adding fiber supplements are all good ways to increase your fiber intake. The fiber to look for is psyllium, which sometimes can cause bloating. Laxatives may be needed, but remember, they can create dependence. Inappropriate use of laxatives can create serious problems, and over time they lose their effectiveness. The least harmful laxatives are stool softeners without stimulants, as opposed to other forms that work by stimulating bowel activity. Severe constipation can lead to bowel impaction. The usual treatment for bowl impaction is a gloved finger in the rectum to feel for hard stool. Obviously, this is unpleasant for everyone involved. But removing impacted stool manually can bring great relief and make subsequent caregiving easier. An enema can break up the impacted stool, but overzealous use of enemas may create its own problems.

Insomnia

Older people often seem to sleep less. Sometimes the sleep cycle changes with age. An older person may spend fewer hours sleeping at night, and offset this by taking naps during the day. This napping can make it harder to fall asleep at night. There are also a number of physiological causes for insomnia in older people. Shortness of breath from a heart condition, for instance, can cause someone to wake up. So, too, can pain. Pulmonary problems, sometimes called sleep apnea, can cause a similar problem. Things like restless leg syndrome, anxiety, and depression can also keep someone up at night. In institutions, getting to sleep may be hard because lights are left on or noises in the corridor are disconcerting. And during room checks, patients in hospitals and some nursing homes are woken up "to see if they are sleeping." Older people can also have trouble sleeping simply because they wake up frequently during the night to use the bathroom. In this case, it can be hard to tell the cart from the horse. Do they wake up because they need to go to the bathroom or do they go to the bathroom because they are already awake?

Sleep Medications

Older people often expect to use a medication to get more sleep, but these drugs can be harmful. Some are specifically discouraged (see the section on drugs on page 163 for more information on what to avoid). Narcotics, for example, can cause balance problems, which lead to higher rates of falls. Sleeping medications can also cause daytime drowsiness and confusion, and they can be addictive. Many sleeping problems can be managed by behavioral conditioning and common sense. Lots of exercise, fewer naps, consistent bedtime routines, few or no caffeinated beverages, and avoiding liquids before bedtime are good ways to foster sleep without resorting to drugs.

Depression

Age is no protection against mental illness. Certainly it is unlikely that an older person will develop a new major psychosis. But people with severe mental illness do reach old age and older people can suffer from new mental health problems. If an older person does develop a new mental health problem, chances are high that it will be depression. About 10 percent of elderly people living outside of nursing homes suffer from depression and the rates are considerably higher among nursing home residents. This depression can be situational (associated with loss or other traumas) or primary (not related to any other event or problem). Depression is the most common psychiatric problem in older people, much more prevalent than dementia. It is often treatable, but unfortunately it is also often overlooked or misdiagnosed. Many of the traditional physical signs of depression like loss of appetite, fatigue, and trouble sleeping are dismissed as typical problems with older people.

Recognizing Depression

Major clinical depression warrants active antidepressant medications. The challenge is to distinguish clinical depression from less severe forms of depression and other problems that mimic depression, like sadness, frustration, and grief. Depression may be a stand-alone problem, or it may also occur alongside other problems, including Alzheimer's disease, stroke, and other forms of dementia. Depression can complicate recovery from many illnesses, especially if it manifests in complaints about intractable pain.

Symptoms that look like depression can actually just be responses to trying situations. As people get older, they are more subject to various types of losses—spouses, friends, pets, driving, sight, mobility—than the rest of us. Grieving can mimic depression or serve as a trigger for the development of a depressive episode. Even the loss of a driver's license can lead older persons to feel unhappy and showing many signs of depressed behavior. This means that the cardinal signs of depression (shown in Table 6.1) can be easily ignored by both the older person and family members. Both may simply dismiss these signs as a reaction to a loss or a consequence of old age. Like many areas of geriatrics, distinguishing normal age-related changes from pathologic changes (those caused by a disease) is a challenge.

When it comes to depression, it is probably best to err on the side of caution. If symptoms persist for more than several weeks, they should be investigated.

If Table 6.1 indicates that depression is likely, you might want to look at the Geriatric Depression Scale, which is the basic test for depression. It is

Table 6.1: Depressive Symptoms

If a person has at least three of the following symptoms for more than two weeks, their condition should be investigated.
Persistent sadness
Crying
Feelings of hopelessness
Persistent anxiety
Weight loss
Sleep disturbances
Loss of energy
Unexplained pain
Loss of appetite
Lack of interest in activities
Frequent and prolonged napping
Difficulty concentrating
Suicidal thoughts

reproduced in Table 6.2, although I have found that a single question—"Are you feeling sad or blue?"—can readily identify people who need to be investigated for depression.

To score the test, give 1 point for every *yes* answer except for questions marked with an asterisk; for those, give 1 point for each *no*. A score greater than 5 suggests depression. A score greater than 10 almost always indicates depression and is grounds for a referral for professional treatment.

Table 6.2: Geriatric Depression Scale

Respondent should choose the best answer for each question that describes how he or she felt over the past week. Each question should be answered *yes* or *no*.	
1.	Are you basically satisfied with life?*
2.	Have you dropped many of your activities and interests?
3.	Do you feel that your life is empty?
4.	Do you often get bored?
5.	Are you in good spirits most of the time?*
6.	Are you afraid that something bad may happen to you?
7.	Do you feel happy most of the time?*
8.	Do you often feel helpless?
9.	Do you prefer to stay at home, rather than going out and doing new things?
10.	Do you feel you have more problems with memory than most?
11.	Do you think it is wonderful to be alive now?*
12.	Do you feel pretty worthless the way you are now?
13.	Do you feel full of energy?*
14.	Do you feel your situation is hopeless?
15.	Do you think that most people are better off than you are?

Source: J. A. Yesavage and T. L. Brink, "Development and Validation of a Geriatric Depression Screening Scale: A Preliminary Report," *Journal of Psychiatric Research* 17, no. 1 (1983): 37–49.

Depression Medications

Depression is caused by chemical imbalances in the brain involving neurotransmitters such as serotonin, norepinephrine, and dopamine. A number of different medications are available to treat depression. They all go by the title "antidepressants," but they work quite differently. The newer drugs affect the brain's uptake of serotonin. The most commonly prescribed class of drugs, called selective serotonin reuptake inhibitors, or SSRIs (such as Prozac, Zoloft, and Paxil), work by inhibiting serotonin uptake. Tricyclics (such as Nefazodone) are an older method of treating depression. They work by inhibiting serotonin and norepinephrine uptake in the brain. Trazodone works on serotonin uptake as well, and bupropion (sold under the name Wellbutrin) weakly inhibits brain cells' use of norepinephrine, serotonin, and dopamine. Monoamine oxidase inhibitors, or MAOIs, increase the levels of neurotransmitters by affecting the chemicals that metabolize them. These are very rarely prescribed, however, because they interact dangerously with common foods.

The biggest factor in choosing the best drug is the prescribing doctor's experience with that drug. It is often safer and better for a physician to work with the drugs he or she knows best, rather than adopting each widely advertised new product.

Prescription Drugs

Older people are often drug addicts; they take a lot of drugs. People over sixty-five make up about 15 percent of the population, but they use more than 35 percent of all prescribed medications. At least 90 percent of elderly people take at minimum one prescribed medication daily. On average, older people take three to eight drugs daily, both prescribed and over the counter (OTC). Some older adults take anywhere from nine to twenty-four different drugs each day. Older people respond to drugs differently from younger people. It is easier to overmedicate older patients for several reasons:

- Body composition changes with age—there is more fat and less muscle. Some drugs are water soluble and others fat soluble. Fat-soluble drugs will be stored for long periods and hence be around even after the drug is discontinued.
- Less body mass means less space for the drug to distribute and hence higher concentrations in older people.
- Many drugs have an active and inactive form in the body. The inactive form binds to body proteins, which may be less available in older people. This means more of the drug remains in the active form longer.
- Some drugs are metabolized (rendered inactive) in the liver. Older people may have decreased liver function, which makes them less able to metabolize the drugs as quickly.
- Some drugs are excreted by the kidneys. Most older people have reduced kidney function, so they cannot excrete the drug as quickly.

The upshot is that drugs may have more potent effects on older people. They hang around longer in the body, so levels of medication can build up. Because of this, great care must be taken when prescribing medications for older people. The general geriatric rule of thumb is "start low, go slow." The initial dosages prescribed can be lower than the levels recommended for younger adults and should be increased gradually. The prescribing doctor should carefully monitor their patients' blood levels and pay attention to potential side effects. (Remember that just as with new symptoms of a disease, side effects are harder to recognize in older people, who already have lots of other medical problems.)

Multiple Medications in Combination Increases Overdosing Risk

Obviously, the more pills an older person is taking, the higher his risk of overmedication. Many older people take dozens of pills to address their many illnesses. The average older person takes at least five pre-scribed drugs, not to mention over-the-counter medications and herbal pills and supplements. Many elderly people are literally walking chemis-try sets, full of drugs that can interact with each other or with one of their other conditions. Sometimes older people are inadvertently taking mul-tiple drugs of the same type. Each physician prescribes a drug she thinks is needed without checking to see what is already in play, or she may fail to adequately instruct the patient to stop one drug when they start another. Caregivers must be vigilant about potential duplicated prescrip-tions or drug classes. That is why it is important to keep a medication list as recommended in Chapter Three.

Finding the right drug dosage is an important skill. It requires systematic observation of the intended effects as well as the side effects of the drugs. The geriatrician's drug axiom is start low, go slow. Because older people don't metabolize drugs as well, they can build up high levels quickly and often in an active form. A patient's regi-men may need to be adjusted regularly. Physicians need direct observa-tions about how well the drugs are working. Because our current health care system makes it difficult and unrewarding for physicians to monitor their patients on that level, family members need to step in. As discussed in the section on caregiving, if you learn what to look for, you can accu-rately track the effectiveness of the different drugs your care recipient is taking.

Multiple Medication Regimens Can Be Confusing

Just as multiple medications increase risk of overmedication, they also increase the risk of messing up a prescribed regimen. It is easy to confuse one drug with another or to mix up the timing schedule. If an older per-son is taking twelve different medications, how is she supposed to keep straight which ones should be taken with food and which ones should not? Fortunately, systems are available to help people avoid mistakes.

There are pill boxes that organize medications by day and dosage time or pre-sealed plastic bags containing single doses for each dosage period. There are also special pill bottles with computer chips in the cap to record when the bottle has been opened so that a person can be sure she won't accidentally take the same pill twice. There are even pill bottles available with reminder alarms that beep or flash when it is time to take a pill. A low-tech option is to put the pill bottle upside down or to put a coin on the cup each time a dose is taken.

Administering Medications

Caregivers and anyone supervising the care of older people should know how their medications should be administered. Although many older people may want their drugs to be crushed and dissolved in food, not all drugs can be taken this way. Make sure to ask your physician or pharmacist if this is an option. Some drugs react to certain foods and lose their effectiveness. Each prescription's label should tell you if the drug should be taken on an empty stomach. A more common problem is that doctors and pharmacists sometimes forget to warn about drugs that cannot be taken with certain foods. So remember to ask specifically about any foods that should be avoided.

It is critical to understand just how the medications are meant to be taken. That is harder to do than it seems. Even skilled and patient doctors and pharmacists who take the time to explain how to take the drugs do not always make things clear. Most people do not understand common instructions for taking drugs. Stop and think for a minute what is meant by taking a pill three times a day. When should it be taken? Is three times a day different from every eight hours? When should you wake up to take your medicine? What does it mean not to take a pill with meals? How long should you wait after eating? How long before a meal can you take it? What do you do if you miss a dose? Double up next time? Just skip it?

Cost-Saving Strategies

Some medications are very expensive. Occasionally it is possible to halve the cost by a double dosage being prescribed and cutting the pills in half. If you are curious about this strategy, make sure to talk to your prescribing physician or a pharmacist before you start chopping. Some pills, like timed-release capsules, cannot be safely cut. If you get your physician's okay, and do opt to pursue this route for your parent, a pill cutter is a necessity.

But if an older person cannot afford the pills, it is not better to take half a dose. It is critical to discuss financial strain and affordability of medications with the doctor. Otherwise you are all acting out a charade where he pretends to prescribe them and the older person promises to take them. In many instances much cheaper generic drugs can be substituted.

Dangerous Drugs

Certain drugs are especially dangerous for older people. Table 6.3 lists those drugs. Table 6.4 provides examples of drugs that shouldn't be taken if you suffer from certain medical conditions. Table 6.5 shows drugs that exacerbate the effects of other drugs and should not be taken together. None of these lists is complete and should be used with care. Sometimes one of these drugs is truly needed. It is always good to talk with your prescribing physician or a pharmacist about any concerns.

Sometimes certain drugs can exacerbate or even produce the symptoms of a disease or condition. For example, the following drugs may exacerbate or mimic dementia:

- Anticholinergics (e.g., diphenhydramine, amitriptyline)
- Sedatives/hypnotics (e.g., benzodiazepines)
- Skeletal muscle relaxants (e.g., carisoprodol [Soma], methocarbamol [Robaxin], cyclobenzaprine [Flexeril], baclofen [Lioresal])
- Opioids (e.g., Darvon, Darvocet)
- Steroids

Similarly, a number of drug types can increase the risk of falls:

- Ambien
- Antidepressants
- Antiepileptics
- Antipsychotics
- Benzodiazepines
- Opioids (especially new start)

Table 6.3: Medications Elders Should Stay Away From

Amiodarone
Anticholinergics (amitriptyline, olanzapine, paroxetine, diphenhydramine (e.g., Tylenol PM, Advil PM)
Benzodiazepines
Digoxin
Fluoxetine
Glyburide
Meperidine
Nitrofurantoin
NSAIDs
Opioids (e.g., propoxyphene and acetaminophen, fentanyl)
Skeletal muscle relaxants (e.g., cyclobenzaprine, carisoprodol, methocarbamol)

Sources: D. M. Fick, et al., Archives of Internal Medicine 163 (2003): 2716–24.
ACOVE criteria. E. L. Knight, et al., Annals of Internal Medicine 135 (2001): 703–10.
Clinical Management System regulations (nursing homes).
M. L. Chew, et al., Journal of the American Geriatrics Society 56 (2008): 133–41.

Table 6.4: Medications and Diseases That Don't Get Along

Disease	Medications to Avoid
Epilepsy	Clozapine (Clozaril), chlorpromazine, thioridazine, chlorprothixene, Metoclopramide
Insomnia	Decongestants Theophylline Desipramine, serotonin selective reuptake inhibitors (SSRIs), monoamine oxidase inhibitors (MAOIs) Beta-agonists
Constipation	Anticholinergics Opiates Tricyclic antidepressants
Ulcers	NSAIDs Aspirin Potassium supplements
Diabetes	Beta blockers Corticosteroids
Asthma	Beta blockers
Chronic obstructive pulmonary disease	Beta blockers Sedative hypnotics
Arrhythmias	Tricyclic antidepressants
Heart failure	Disopyramide Drugs with high sodium content
Blood clotting disorders being treated with anticoagulants	Aspirin
Hypertension	Amphetamines
Peripheral vascular disease	Beta blockers
Syncope	Beta blockers Long-acting benzodiazepines

Table 6.4 (continued)

Disease	Medications to Avoid
Benign prostate hypertrophy	Anticholinergic antihistamines Anticholinergic antidepressants Gastrointestinal antispasmodics Muscle relaxants Narcotics (including propoxyphene) Flavoxate, oxybutynin Bethanechol (Urecholine)
Incontinence Impaired mental status	Alpha blockers Beta blockers, psychoactive medications

Table 6.5: High-Risk Drug Combinations

Warfarin
NSAIDs (e.g., ibuprofen)
Antiplatelets
Trimethoprim-sulfamethoxazole (Bactrim, Septra)
Erythromycin, clarithromycin (Biaxin)
Quinolones (e.g., Cipro, Levaquin, Avelox)
Phenytoin (Dilantin)
Digoxin
Amiodarone
Verapamil (Calan)
ACE inhibitors (e.g., lisinopril)/Angiotensin receptor blockers (e.g., Diovan, "-sartans")
Potassium supplements
Spironolactone (Aldactone)
Potassium-sparing agents (Dyazide, Maxzide)

Table 6.5 (continued)

Trimethoprim (e.g., Bactrim, Septra)
NSAIDs
Theophylline (e.g., Theo-24, Uniphyl, others)
Quinolones
Quinolones
Calcium, iron, aluminum, magnesium, zinc
Enteral feeding products

Source: Drug interaction resource: http://medicine.iupui.edu/flockhart.

Communication About Medications Is Essential

None of these lists is complete; they are sets of general rules. The lists should be used to raise alerts in discussing medications with physicians and pharmacists. Sometimes there might be an exception. One of these medications may be necessary to the care of an older person. However, it never hurts to ask about alternatives. Great caution should be used every time a patient begins taking a new drug. Family members should be prepared to ask the prescribing physician if the drug appears on one of these lists, and if it will have negative interactions with any of the other drugs the patient is currently taking.

In many cases, it is better to talk to the pharmacist, who might know more about the actual composition of the prescribed drug and may be more willing to discuss drug-related issues. Many pharmacists, especially in drugstore chains, have developed computerized systems that scan new prescriptions to look for potential duplications and adverse interactions with drugs already prescribed. (It offers patients an inducement to fill all their prescriptions in one place.) Warnings are generated that alert the pharmacist to discuss these potential events with the prescribing doctor. Sometimes they will even tell the patient, but you should ask about these.

Be Cautious About Sedation

You will probably face strong pressures to allow your loved one to be put on drugs to be sedated or calmed. Residents of institutions are more easily managed when they are sedated. But these medications are potent. Many older people are already taking several medications on any given day, and sedating or calming drugs might interact with existing medications. Additionally, these drugs can decrease a person's quality of life and may be dangerous in their own right. Use of sedatives can lead to falls, accidents, and even some disease complications (see Table 6.4). They can complicate or induce mental confusion. Excessive use of sleeping medications can actually interfere with sleep, as well as become addictive.

Psychoactive Drugs and Dementia: Know the Risks and Realities

Our society is quick to medicate. One of the greatest temptations is to use psychoactive drugs to control the behavior of people with dementia. Their behavior can be hard to deal with, and can be seen as threatening to themselves and disruptive to others. However, a recent study has shown that antipsychotic medications can produce more harm than good. There is no strong evidence that prescribing psychoactive drugs to control the behavior of dementia patients is appropriate, and most experts will warn against this use. If behaviorally disruptive people with dementia are medicated to the point of silence, their behavior may become consistent with that of people suffering from some psychoses. Obviously, you want to avoid this. Before medicating, other means of management should be actively tried.

Challenges of Nonpharmacological Behavior Management

Fair warning, though: finding nonpharmacological ways to address disruptive behaviors can be a caregiver's greatest challenge. Experts who study this have put forward various strategies for dealing with disruptive behavior. Most of these require substantial time one-on-one with patients to observe and to interact with them. You need to understand what triggers a rage reaction and how to avoid such behaviors. Some basic techniques are straightforward, but just as with parenting, it requires patience and persistence. Most care systems don't provide care with that level of attention, and will push for a pharmacological form of behavior control. This continues today, even as medical literature is waking up to what geriatricians have known for years—drugs should be used only as a last resort.

Finding a Middle Ground

Families of dementia patients may find themselves in a difficult bind. When organizing care for my own mother, we were caught between two difficult alternatives. The staff at her assisted-living facility insisted that unless an active and substantial intervention was put in place, she would have to be transferred to a nursing home. But psychoactive drugs were as likely to exacerbate her condition as to improve it, and we were concerned that the drugs would cause falls. Ultimately, we went through several cycles of medication treatment and withdrawal, struggling to find a middle ground. It is very hard to avoid psychoactive medications unless the caregivers (family or staff) are truly committed to trying.

If a dementia patient is put on psychoactive drugs, it is essential that everyone involved in caring for that person monitor the situation closely. Everyone needs to be ready to report any significant change—for better or for worse. The prescribing doctor must oversee the situation and adjust dosages accordingly. Getting everyone on board and working in harmony is no easy task, but it is well worth the effort. Ideally the staffs of nursing homes, and hopefully assisted-living facilities, have been trained on how to work with residents with challenging behavior. This training should cover what actions can trigger outbursts and how staff attitudes and behavior can affect the client's behavior.

How to Handle Pain

Pain can play a major role in the lives of older persons. And unfortunately, it is often poorly managed. Too many older people suffer from chronic and intractable pain, often related to osteoarthritis. Most of the time, this pain can be alleviated or at least managed. Pain-relieving medications (analgesics) come in many forms. Strong drugs require a doctor's prescription, but many milder and still effective forms don't. Also, there are ways to manage pain without analgesics. Other types of treatments like meditation, massage, and acupuncture can help to prevent or reduce pain. For some people, these methods can be equally or even more effective than drugs.

Analgesics for Pain Prevention

One of the biggest myths about pain management is that analgesics should be given in response to pain. Somehow, we have all started believing that analgesia must be earned through suffering. There is a better way. Lower doses of drugs can be used to prevent, or at least minimize pain, compared to what it takes to respond to it. It may require some experimentation to find the most effective dosage and dosing schedule. But it is worth it. The best way to cope with chronic pain is to identify the lowest dose that will prevent pain or keep it at a level that allows the older person to cope. It may not be possible to eliminate pain altogether, but it is almost always possible to keep it at a tolerable level. A nurse or doctor may ask you, "On a scale of one to ten, with ten being the worst pain you can imagine, how bad is your pain?" Once your pain level reaches six or seven, it's harder to manage. More medication is required and it is much more difficult for you to function. Obviously, every person has their own basis for their pain scales, but the goal should always be to keep pain below a five.

How to Choose the Right Analgesic

There are a broad range of analgesics with a wide variety of strengths and side effects. As you may recall, older patients run a serious risk of being overmedicated. In elder care, the line between too little and too much treatment is usually thin. A delicate balance must be struck between over- and underprescribing pain relievers. It is best to start with the least toxic types of medication, and to avoid opiates and synthetic opiates as long as possible.

Aspirin and Tylenol

Even over-the-counter analgesics like aspirin and acetaminophen (aka Tylenol) can have serious side effects. Aspirin can cause stomach upset and bleeding. Many people can tolerate those symptoms, especially if they take antacids with the aspirin. However, taking pain medication and antacids at the same time is not recommended. Aspirin use also increases the likelihood that you could suffer very serious GI bleeding without preceding gastric discomfort. Once again, age increases your risk. Luckily, if this kind of severe GI bleeding is going to occur, it usually does so soon after you begin using aspirin. Acetaminophen can have side effects. Common problems include difficulties metabolizing sugar (glucose) and reduced liver function, so be sure to keep an eye out for warning signs.

Just as with prescribed pain medications, the goal should be to find the lowest effective dose. Once you've done that, you can use that dose proactively to prevent the pain. A good way to prevent excessive use of aspirin or acetaminophen can be to alternate. For example, one could take Tylenol at noon and aspirin at 6 p.m.

Nonsteroidal Anti-Inflammatory Drugs: Motrin, Advil, and Others

Nonsteroidal anti-inflammatory drugs (NSAIDs) are another type of analgesics. NSAIDs include ibuprofen (sold over the counter as Motrin and Advil) and a number of prescription medications. NSAIDs carry their own risk profiles. Ibuprofen can damage both the kidneys and the intestines, and should not be used by anyone facing declining kidney function. It can also cause edema (or swelling of the feet). NSAIDs should not be taken at the same time as aspirin because both types of drugs can damage the GI tract and have a greater negative effect when taken together. Not only that, but when used together, pain relief actually goes down. If a person uses aspirin for heart problems and takes a NSAID for pain relief, these two doses should be separated by at least twenty minutes to ensure that each medication is as effective as possible. COX-2 selective inhibitors are the newest class of NSAIDs, and concerns about these drugs are growing. There have been reports of increased risks to the heart. One of these drugs, rofecoxib (Vioxx), has already been pulled off the market by its manufacturer. People who take NSAIDs regularly should take some form of antacid like a proton pump inhibitor (e.g., omeprazole).

Opiates

Opiates should not be used to relieve mild pain, but they can be very helpful for managing severe pain or pain that interferes with function (ADLs and IADLs). The careful use of opiates, both in the short-term and in the long-term, can increase mobility and the ability to rehabilitate. Opiates do carry an increased risk of sedation and falling, but can greatly improve quality of life when appropriately used. There is an irrational fear that prescribing opiates will create a generation of elderly dope addicts. In fact, opiates have been used effectively to manage pain in older people and should be considered as part of the larger repertoire, after more basic approaches have been tried. It is certainly foolish to keep someone in pain for fear of creating an addiction.

Delirium

Hospitals are dangerous places for sick old people. Anyone transforming into the role of a hospital patient pays a big price. They give up their identity, familiar things, even their privacy. They have to wear gaping gowns. Their routines are subordinated to those of the institution. (For more on the dangers of hospitals, see Chapter Eight.)

People who are hospitalized are, clearly, sick or injured. The stress of hospitalization can compound this. Placing a vulnerable person in a stressful environment is a ticket to disaster. For an older patient, treatment for many conditions is essentially a series of stressful activities. Combine that with the introduction of substances like anesthetics and strong drugs, and it is hardly surprising that older patients frequently become confused and disoriented during hospital stays. Acute instances of confusion are called delirium. Delirium should always be promptly and actively investigated. Sometimes delirium is an early indication of dementia. But most times, if the underlying problem is promptly and correctly treated, delirium is reversible. However, even with treatment, the effects of delirium may persist for some time.

Recognizing Delirium

It can be tough to recognize delirium for what it is when it first occurs. One of the difficulties is that delirium can be caused by many different things: oxygen deprivation, infection, anesthesia, sedatives, indwelling catheters, dehydration, psychoactive drugs, or metabolic imbalances. Not all physicians or nurses catch it soon enough. They may dismiss delirium as the result of simple age-related problems and allow it to run its course, untreated. This is bad! Delirium is a major threat to an older person's health. If left untreated, it can have serious permanent consequences.

Distinguishing Delirium from Dementia

Although the two conditions share symptoms, it is very important to distinguish delirium from dementia. Dementia develops gradually. Delirium, on the other hand, is an acute state of confusion. It is often brought on by a metabolic event; anesthesia, for example, or a change in the blood levels of electrolytes such as sodium and potassium. If treated early, delirium is usually reversible. Dementia is not.

Table 6.6: Symptoms of Delirium

Acute change in mental status (onset of confusion, loss of faculties)
Fluctuating course
Attention disturbance (unable to stay focused on a topic or idea)
Memory disturbance
Orientation disturbance (does not know time, place, or person)
Perceptual disturbance (does not see, hear, or interpret things correctly)
Disorganized or incoherent thinking (has strange ideas, may be paranoid, suspicious)
Sleep disturbance (can't fall asleep)
Consciousness disturbance (can't stay awake)
Speech disturbance
Psychomotor activity disturbance (starts to get agitated and moves around)

Persons with dementia can also suffer from delirium. In fact, one condition aggravates the other. The major symptoms of delirium are shown in Table 6.6.

Tools for Detecting Delirium

Because delirium can be difficult to recognize, specific screening tools are available to help doctors and nurses detect the condition. One of the best is the Confusion Assessment Method (CAM). The CAM assesses four markers of delirium: a sudden and severe change or an ongoing series of changes in a patient's mental status, inattention, disorganized thinking, and a decreased level of consciousness. If a patient shows signs of a change in mental status and inattention, *and* either disorganized thinking *or* an altered level of consciousness, then it is very likely that patient is suffering from delirium.

To determine the likelihood of delirium, the Confusion Assessment Method uses a series of questions:

1. [Acute onset] Is there evidence of an acute change in mental status from the patient's baseline?

2. [Inattention] Did the patient have difficulty focusing attention, for example, being easily distractible or having difficulty keeping track of what was said? If so, did this behavior fluctuate during the interview, that is, come and go or increase and decrease in severity?

3. [Disorganized thinking] Was the patient's thinking disorganized or incoherent, such as rambling or irrelevant conversation, unclear or illogical flow of ideas, or unpredictably switching from subject to subject?

4. [Altered level of consciousness] Overall, how would you rate the patient's level of consciousness? Alert (normal), vigilant (hyperalert, overly sensitive to environmental stimuli, startles easily), lethargic (drowsy, easily aroused), stupor (difficult to arouse), coma (unarousable).

5. [Disorientation] Was the patient disoriented at any time during the interview, such as thinking that she or he was somewhere other than the hospital, using the wrong bed, or misjudging the time of day?

6. [Memory impairment] Did the patient demonstrate any memory problems during the interview, such as inability to remember events in the hospital or difficulty remembering instructions?

7. [Perceptual disturbances] Did the patient have any evidence of perceptual disturbances; for example, hallucinations, illusions, or misinterpretations (such as thinking something was moving when it was not)?

8. [Psychomotor agitation] At any time during the interview did the patient have an unusually increased level of motor activity,

such as restlessness, picking at bedclothes, tapping fingers, or making frequent sudden changes in position?

9. [Psychomotor retardation] At any time during the interview did the patient have an unusually decreased level of motor activity, such as sluggishness, staring into space, staying in one position for a long time, or moving very slowly?

10. [Altered sleep-wake cycle] Did the patient have evidence of disturbance of the sleep-wake cycle, such as excessive daytime sleepiness with insomnia at night?

Adapted from C. M. Waszynski, "Detecting Delirium," *American Journal of Nursing* 107, no. 12 (2007): 50–59. The CAM material originally appeared in S. Inouye, C. van Dyck, C. Alessi, S. Balkin, A. Siegal, and R. Horwitz, "Clarifying Confusion: The Confusion Assessment Method," *Annals of Internal Medicine* 113, no. 12 (1990): 941–48.

Alcohol

Another mental health issue that can affect older people is alcohol addiction. Late-onset alcoholism is different from alcoholism in younger persons. It is generally more responsive to treatment. Many older people who drink excessively do so in response to their changing situation, including isolation. Because they are not habitual alcoholics, the response to treatment is better if the underlying cause can be addressed.

Alcoholism among older people is often missed. No one likes to think that the sweet little old lady is actually tipsy. Families hesitate to think of their parents as heavy drinkers. But they may well be and the problem will not improve until it is confronted. It is important to look for subtle signs beyond mounds of empty liquor bottles in the trash. Is there increased confusion? Does it occur at certain times that are associated with drinking? Is the older person ordering an extra cocktail?

Chapter Six—Points to Ponder

Aging can mimic illness. Distinguishing between aging and pathology is tough.

Effective treatments do exist. Many diseases of old age can be effectively managed if they are recognized.

Diseases present differently in older persons. The classic symptoms and signs may not apply.

Hip fractures can be fatal. Even when they are not fatal, they are certainly life-changing.

Osteoporosis can be treated. But not every older person needs treatment.

Older people are like walking chemistry sets. They are taking multiple medications, which can interact with each other to cause untoward events. It is very important to keep careful track of what medications an older person is taking and to be sure that every doctor knows what has already been prescribed before adding another drug.

Be attentive for subtle signs of depression. Depression left untreated is at least as dangerous for an older person as for a younger person.

Be attentive for subtle signs of alcoholism. The elderly alcoholic does not resemble the familiar younger stereotype.

Seven

The Aging Brain

Frailty creeps in on silent feet. It can be hard to distinguish between normal signs of aging and early symptoms of serious problems. A change in behavior is one of the best early clues. These changes can be symptoms of many different problems, including early-onset dementia, depression, medication mismanagement, vision or hearing loss, and pain. Apathy, withdrawal, and loss of interest in everyday matters may be signs of something serious. Alternately, they may simply be a coping mechanism. Sometimes focusing on a smaller set of issues and activities can help an older person feel competent and in control of their own life. So what's normal and what's not?

Be Observant of Behavior Changes

Unfortunately, it is not easy to know what behavior changes you should worry about. You might even have difficulty pinpointing a change in behavior. Alzheimer's disease typically presents with a very gradual onset, and is often unrecognized until the disease is quite progressed. Symptoms can come on subtly, and older people are especially good at using social skills to cover the telltale tracks of cognitive changes. They may say things like, "I don't like doing that anymore." "This is a foolish waste of time." "I'm happy just sitting here." Sometimes you begin to realize that things are not getting done. Things your parent used to do just never get accomplished. Sometimes it is things like shopping, cooking, or laundry. You gradually become aware that people who were previously neat and organized are not any longer. They seem to be forgetting things, even getting lost, not paying bills, or having trouble balancing their checkbook. Determining whether a behavior change is cause for concern or not requires that you take time to observe the behavior and to explore other things going on in the older person's life.

Older People Respond to Stress Differently

This time is well spent. A number of problems may appear before long-term care becomes necessary. These problems should be carefully evaluated—both their underlying causes and their implications. As I have said before, the signs of common medical problems often look different for older patients than for younger patients. And it is not simply that an older person may show few or none of the typical responses to a disease; they may show entirely different symptoms. Instead of complaining about chest pain, an older person suffering from a heart attack might become confused. Confusion can also be an older patient's response to pneumonia, rather than the typical fever and cough. However, the same symptom can be a normal result of aging, not an indicator of a disease. A heart attack or pneumonia may be marked by confusion, but something as benign as difficulty in hearing can also make an older person appear confused and disoriented.

Obviously, because something as basic as confusion can be a marker of many different problems, one of the difficulties in caring for older people is correctly determining the origin of their problems. Picking up on early clues increases the chances that proper medical treatment will be able to solve, or at least diminish, the problem.

Strokes

In contrast to dementia, strokes occur suddenly and need prompt attention. When it comes to strokes, prompt recognition of the problem is a key part of successful treatment. Essentially, a stroke is a problem in the arteries in the brain. The technical term is "cerebrovascular accident," or CVA. A stroke can take two forms. Either a clot forms or a bleed occurs. In either case, the brain is damaged.

Different Treatment for Different Stroke Types

However, distinguishing between the two forms of stroke is important because the immediate treatment is very different depending on the type of stroke. Clots are treated with thrombolytic medications designed to dissolve the clot. This treatment would make a bleeding stroke much worse. It is therefore essential to determine right away if the stroke is due to a bleed or a clot. This can be done by using a test called magnetic resonance imaging, or MRI. It is important to do an MRI as soon as possible, because the clot-dissolving medication must be given within three hours of the stroke if it is going to work. This means that if you believe an older

STROKE WARNING SIGNS

The American Stroke Association lists the following warning signs of stroke:

- Sudden numbness or weakness of the face, arm, or leg, especially on one side of the body
- Sudden confusion, or trouble speaking or understanding
- Sudden trouble seeing in one or both eyes
- Pupil sizes are different
- Sudden trouble walking, dizziness, or loss of balance or coordination
- Sudden, severe headache with no known cause

If any of these symptoms occur, and *especially* if more than one occurs, dial 911 immediately!

person is having a stroke, it is crucial to get her to the emergency room immediately, while there is still time to use effective treatments.

What Causes a Stroke?

While there is no certain trigger for a stroke, stroke patients often have hypertension or atrial fibrillation. Saying someone is hypertensive is just a different way of saying that person has high blood pressure. Hypertension can lead to cerebral hemorrhages in the same way that a pipe under great pressure is more likely to burst. Atrial fibrillation refers to an abnormal heartbeat, a condition in which the heart has an abnormally rapid irregular rhythm. This can create clots in the heart that may break loose and go to the brain. Fortunately, both hypertension and atrial fibrillation are treatable.

Drugs used to manage hypertension are called "antihypertensive agents." Chronic atrial fibrillation is usually treated with blood thinners (aka anticoagulants) like Coumadin or heparin, which do not treat the fibrillation but prevent the clots from forming in the heart and flying off. There are also special treatments to convert the abnormal heart rhythm of atrial fibrillation to a more normal rhythm; sometimes they work and sometimes they don't. It is important to be careful when taking antihypertensive agents or anticoagulants. Overtreating or undertreating these conditions is dangerous. Make sure doctor's orders are followed, and check in regularly to make sure treatment is going according to plan. Patients on anticoagulants need to be monitored closely to be sure their clotting time is within an acceptable range. Too high or too low is dangerous.

Recovery After Stroke

The results of a stroke will be different depending on where in the brain the stroke strikes. Generally, a stroke will affect the patient's ability to control different muscles (aka the motor function) and/or her ability to speak. It can also affect sensation. In some cases, the patient can speak but can't communicate intelligibly. That is to say, she is saying words but not making sense. Some speech problems are the result of impaired muscle control, but other problems relate to brain injury. They may have trouble finding the words they want. This is termed "aphasia." Strokes can also affect one's ability to think and reason (aka cognition). After a stroke, thinking may become impulsive and erratic or it may become slow and burdensome. Strokes can also cause memory loss and confusion.

Unlike other brain-function problems that come with old age, strokes do not necessarily lead to permanent changes in brain function. Our brains are programmed to recover from strokes. Most people make full or at least partial recoveries. Good rehabilitation certainly oils the tracks of the recovery process, but it is hard to be sure how much of the gain is due to the body's built-in stroke recovery process and how much is due to the treatment.

Special Stroke Units

The best way to treat a stroke is to be admitted to a special stroke unit. These units are staffed with personnel who are familiar with strokes. If the hospital does not have a stroke unit, they may put older stroke patients in intensive care units (ICUs) where they can receive more intensive nursing. But this noisy, busy area can be a disastrous place for fragile stroke patients. The light, noise, and activity of an ICU can be confusing and overstimulating. My mother was placed in an ICU after her stroke and the overstimulation made her very hard to manage. The danger is that once such a patient gets excited, they will be sedated. Sedation is just what stroke patients do not need; they are already often confused. Sometimes sedatives can have a paradoxical effect; they can make patients more excitable.

Families should ask the doctor—politely—whether the patient could be managed just as well in a less hectic environment. Even if the answer is no, ask the doctor about moving the patient out of the ICU at the earliest possible time.

After the initial thrombolytic treatment to dissolve a clot, not much can be done during the early stages of a stroke. The best way to treat a stroke is to support and stabilize the patient, and to begin rehabilitation as quickly as possible. Early physical therapy can improve the outcome of many strokes. As soon as the patient's condition is stable, he should be transferred to a rehabilitation unit and begin aggressive rehabilitative exercises. More information on rehabilitation can be found in the Rehabilitation section of Chapter Eight.

Dementia

"Dementia" is a general term that is used to describe a chronic loss of mental or cognitive ability. There are many types of dementia, but Alzheimer's disease is by far the most common.

VISITING MOM AFTER ALZHEIMER'S

Dad hardly talks at all, but he loves to listen, or to joke, and he never misses a chance for a pun. Like Shakespeare, he always treated the pun as the very highest form of humor. And Mom still treats his puns with a roll of her eyes, a slight shake of her head, and her inimitable half-smile, half-grimace.

Mom talks and talks, sprinkling her always impressive vocabulary, every word used properly, into improbable monologues to loved ones long gone. I go with her as if on a guided tour of Eden, and I'm whoever, wherever, whenever she needs me to be.

They never want me to leave, but I have to go. We hug and we kiss and we exchange "I love yous" and "See you tomorrows." They walk me to the elevator and we blow kisses and say good-bye long after the door closes.

I never cry when I'm with them, or when I leave them. I'm happy. I had today. I had the chance to make them smile, and I did. I had the chance to hug them, and I did. I had the chance to be with them knowing that we might not have tomorrow, but we had yesterday, and we had today, and that's enough.

—CAROLE HOWEY, CAREGIVING DAUGHTER

Many people are offended by the term "dementia." They prefer to use another term, like "cognitive impairment." I do not think euphemisms help. Dementia can be devastating, both to the person suffering from dementia and to their family. Because that devastation can be so great, softening the term actually does a disservice to everyone involved. No matter what name you use, dementing illnesses will usually affect several aspects of a person's ability to think (in other words, her cognitive function).

Loss of Memory and Executive Function

Memory problems are the most common symptom. Usually the memory loss comes on gradually. It is more likely to affect recent memories than very old ones. Hence persons with dementia may talk a great deal about the past. Because they cannot remember what they have just said, they repeat themselves and can infuriatingly ask the same questions over and over again. Other areas of cognitive performance affected by dementia include so-called executive functions (like making reasoned decisions or interpreting concepts), performing arithmetic calculations, and having a sense of where they are. Getting lost regularly, having trouble with maintaining a checkbook, or starting to forget names can be warning signs of dementia.

The pattern of cognitive function with dementia can vary widely by stage and person. My mother-in-law became severely demented to the point that she was frequently confused about where she was or what was planned, but she could still do a crossword puzzle. My mother suffered from severe dementia but retained her sense of irony and humor long after her memory failed. She might not remember what she had for lunch, but she could phrase an original ironic comment. This inconsistent pattern or performance can make caregiving even more trying if the caregiver cannot judge just how bad the situation is.

Dementia is associated with a number of behaviors that can drive caregivers crazy. Table 7.1 lists the most troublesome behaviors that seem to contribute to most feelings of caregiver burden. All but the last three are also associated with a higher likelihood of nursing home admission.

Table 7.1: Troublesome Behaviors in Dementia

Forgets what day it is
Loses or misplaces things
Dangerous to others
Thinks things are not there
Hides things
Constantly restless
Dangerous to self
Wanders and gets lost
Does embarrassing things
Leaves tasks uncompleted
Trouble recognizing people
Episodes of anger
Suspicious and accusative
Repetitive questions
Destroys property
Relives the past
Constantly talks

Unfortunately, there are no easy ways to deal with many of these irksome behaviors. In some cases distraction will work, at least sometimes, but problems like wandering and aggression can present serious management issues.

Other Diseases Can Exacerbate Dementia

Aspects of dementia may be exacerbated by other underlying diseases. The most common problem is when people with dementia have pain. They may be unable to communicate the problem. Instead they get agitated. For the caregiver, it is not terribly different from interpreting when babies cry. However, the impulse is to address the agitation rather than assessing what may be causing it.

Other physical problems may make dementia symptoms worse. For example, my mother also had congestive heart failure. Inevitably, when her heart disease got worse, so did her dementia. Once you recognize the linkage it is important to pay special attention to controlling the underlying health problem. It will not get rid of the dementia, but it should make managing it easier.

Is It Alzheimer's Disease?

Not all memory loss is dementia. Doctors have created a whole range of titles, like "minimum cognitive impairment" and "benign senescent forgetfulness" to describe syndromes that involve memory loss but fall short of Alzheimer's. Nonetheless, Alzheimer's disease is common and may come on subtly. Ignoring the danger signs will not make the problems go away. It is worth getting a clear diagnosis if you can, and dealing with the problem straight on. There is an active debate about the value of early diagnosis in Alzheimer's disease. Some argue that identifying the problem early allows a person time to make plans and life adjustments. Some hold out the hope that treatments may be more effective in the early stage of the disease, but so far this is more a hope than a reality. The counterargument holds that it is cruel to induce the anxiety associated with diagnosis earlier than necessary. It probably is not a good idea to rush to the doctor the first time an older person forgets a name. As symptoms become obvious (and they are more obvious when you know what to look for), you can take steps to investigate the cause.

Alzheimer's disease is the most common kind of dementia. Other conditions can mimic the symptoms of dementia, including depression, normal pressure hydrocephalus (a blockage in the fluid system of the brain), Parkinson's disease, and even thyroid disease. If you think a loved one may be suffering from dementia, it's certainly worth investigating for treatable causes. But do not become too optimistic; only a small number of dementias are reversible. There are a number of other esoteric causes, but they all carry at least as grim a prognosis. If you convince yourself that it is *not* dementia, then hearing that it is will be that much harder.

Ideally, knowing the actual type of dementia may help caregivers to predict the course of the disease, but many times it is a distinction without a difference. Indeed, the definitive diagnosis is not made until autopsy and even then, it may not be truly definitive. A few types of dementia have distinct (or at least generally distinct) clinical patterns. For example, multi-infarct dementia is more like a series of small strokes, and has a more stair-step clinical pattern, compared to the gradual course of Alzheimer's. Lewy body dementia, a much rarer form, is typically associated with more neurological changes.

Families are often concerned about the genetics of dementia. Some forms are inheritable, and there are genetic tests for these. Because the tests are not 100 percent accurate in predicting who will get dementia, genetic counseling is strongly recommended (in some clinics required).

KNOWING WHAT'S COMING

Once Mom was evaluated, even though she did not yet have a diagnosis of Alzheimer's disease, we knew it was coming and we were able to prepare. The guiding principles for us were to keep Mom safe and happy, and to be able to reassure her that everything was going to be all right. Maybe Mom's anxiety was just a phase, but it did seem that once the family was all on the same page, once we had agreed how to proceed, and as long as we continued to discuss issues before they became problems, Mom was no longer anxious.

Years after Mom was evaluated and shortly before she moved from her own home into assisted living, a friend of hers stopped me to say how sad it was to see her decline. I thought, "What are you talking about? Mom's doing great! She has no complaints. She's happy. She's safe. Her family is together and supportive of her and each other."

—RILEY McCARTEN, CAREGIVING SON

What You Need to Know About Dementia

Different kinds of dementia will develop in different ways. The pattern of the disease's onset can provide clues to physicians trying to determine the disease's origin (aka its etiology). For example, Alzheimer's disease has a slow and insidious onset. Multi-infarct dementia, however, is caused by a series of small strokes, and therefore develops in a clear step-by-step pattern. In any case, it may take a while before family members recognize that something has changed and is seriously wrong. If you suspect something is awry, it is a good idea to schedule an evaluation for your loved one.

Specialty Medical Centers for Dementia

There are medical clinics that specialize in dementia. These centers are often associated with large academic medical centers. Although a visit may involve some travel and inconvenience, it is worth it. You deserve to get a definitive opinion on your loved one's mental status, and at the very least, some tips for coping with the problem. The multidisciplinary experts at these centers will test for treatable causes and can train caregivers to better cope with persons with dementia. But be realistic. Cures for dementia are scarce.

Anticholinergic Drugs for Dementia

We do not yet have an effective way to treat most dementias. Some doctors will recommend anticholinergic drugs. These drugs increase the availability of the chemicals that facilitate communication between brain cells. They are most effective in the early stages of the disease. While this may sound promising, these drugs are only moderately helpful in slowing the rate of decline. Some optimistic studies suggest you may gain an extra six months of function, but the preponderance of evidence so far is less positive. More often than not, a medication is recommended because experts feel pressure from families to do something. There is still a lot of debate about just how helpful such treatment can be, but dealing with dementia is so stressful that both professionals and families will clutch at every straw. Feel free to ask to the doctors how helpful they truly think the treatment will be.

CAUTION! Dementia specialty clinics may feel under special pressure to offer treatment because that is their raison d'être. Therefore, paradoxically, an older person with dementia may be at a greater risk of getting a medication of questionable value from people who should know better.

You can use a number of strategies to more effectively manage someone with dementia. (Some good resources are provided in the appendix.) You can learn to cope with aggressive behaviors and how to deal with wandering. Memory aids, like memory boards and event calendars, can be useful. Pictures have been shown to help patients remember and relate to people, places, and events.

Caregiving and Dementia

Make no mistake: Taking care of persons with dementia is very hard work. It is probably the most demanding form of caregiving. The person you're caring for may not look like she needs help, but her needs can be daunting and her behavior can be trying. A person with dementia will often repeat the same questions and observations. Understandably, this can grate on caregivers' nerves and keep friends and family from visiting or helping out. And on the flip side, having to repeat directions over and over for your care recipient can be exasperating. But the rewards of caring for an older loved one with dementia can be surprisingly profound. One group of researchers pointed out that although almost all the caregivers of persons with dementia found caregiving stressful, 78 percent found they were able to infuse these times with meaning and joy. They described "bonds that would otherwise not be there."

Emotional Toll of Dementia Caregiving

Caring for someone with dementia can take a very heavy emotional toll. It is no coincidence that the most widely read book on this subject is called *The 36-Hour Day*, by Nancy Mace and Peter Rabins. This aptly titled book was one of the first to really address the unique difficulties of caring for someone with Alzheimer's, a topic that definitely requires solid

A CALM, SLOW APPROACH

You hear many stories about the behavior of individuals with Alzheimer's. One of the things that one has to think about is that a confused person cannot identify people and when someone comes toward the person, they feel threatened. When a person is grabbed to assist them to get out of a chair they feel threatened and occasionally lash out. The usual response to this is that the staff member gets another person to assist them. Now the individual with Alzheimer's feels even more threatened and fights harder. I suggest using a calm, slow approach with the person. It is how I want to be treated. I also found that I got a better response from the elderly if I called them by their title. Men especially responded to being addressed as "Mr." or even "Dr."

—JOANN HOWITZ, CAREGIVER AND PHYSICAL THERAPIST

and honest information for caregivers. Many describe dementia as the worst disease to care for because the person you knew seems to have disappeared even while they are still there. Some people describe it as having the person die while they're still alive. You are left with artifacts of the person they used to be. Dementia goes through stages. Each stage requires different coping skills and knowledge of effective interventions. Support groups can help, but caregivers need more than support. They need instruction in practical and effective ways to care for dementia patients.

There are specific techniques you can use to keep dementia patients calm and to avoid rage reactions. There are also strategies to help families handle the stress of caring for dementia patients. Although it was published in 1981, The *36-Hour Day* is still one of the best resources available, and new editions are available. Local chapters of the Alzheimer's Association can provide useful advice and support, and other references are listed in the appendix. However, no matter how many techniques and strategies and support systems you use, caring for someone with dementia is going to require incredible amounts of patience and love.

A DAUGHTER'S STORY OF DEALING
WITH ALZHEIMER'S

In December 2003, my eighty-three-year-old mother called me in distress the night before she was to arrive for her Christmas visit, claiming she had missed her flight. I reassured her that she had not missed her flight, that she was not due until the following day. This was the first sign that my mother was suffering from Alzheimer's disease. It has been downhill ever since. After her visit, I called her physician and explained her symptoms. He had her tested and in January 2004 diagnosed Alzheimer's. That summer, when my mother, who loved her home, a small colonial abutting a public golf course, admitted to me that she was lonely and that it would perhaps be best if she moved into the Presbyterian retirement community in town where so many of her friends lived, but which she for years had adamantly referred to as "the home," a place to which she would never move, I jumped and immediately made an appointment with the admissions director. Less than six weeks later, a deluxe apartment was available and we took it. My sister and I spent days cleaning out thirty years of accumulation in our mother's home, filling a Dumpster and more. Mom kept berating us, pulling suitcases and pots and pans out of the Dumpster, insisting that these things represented her life and that she needed them and how could we possibly throw them away?

We soldiered on, and in the fall of 2004 moved Mom into a two-bedroom, two-bathroom apartment in the independent living building of the Presbyterian home. It was a nightmare. Mom had a yellow legal pad on which she had written copious notes about various items from the house. Frenetically, she flipped from page to page, asking about the whereabouts of the cameras in the sideboard drawers, Grandma and Grandpa's sugar bowl, the silver platter that was her mother's. She was beside herself and just kept repeating her concerns over and over. At one point I returned from an errand to find my sister in tears, saying, "I can't take this anymore . . . promise me, if I ever am like this, you will shoot me." I agreed.

As Mom's Alzheimer's progressed, we fought about caregivers, but she has long since acquiesced. Since 2004, she has suffered several strokes and is basically bedridden and does not know who we are. We are blessed to have several wonderful caregivers and her financial situation is such that she does not have to worry.

—CAREGIVING DAUGHTER

Chapter Seven—Points to Ponder

Acute confusion is different from dementia. Acute confusion is a common symptom that can have many causes. It should be carefully evaluated.

Delirium is a life-threatening condition. It should not be ignored or dismissed.

Good stroke care makes a big difference.

Dementia is hard to deal with. We do not have effective treatments. It takes a heavy toll on caregivers. There are ways to cope more effectively.

Have warning signs checked out early. It is worth evaluating a person with persistent signs of confusion and memory impairment.

But not too early. It is probably not worth launching such an evaluation prematurely. The key is to establish that the signs are persistent, not isolated or extremely occasional incidents.

There is no cure. No good treatments for Alzheimer's disease are yet available. There is a great temptation to use drugs because they may do some good. Be realistic.

Eight

Handling Hospitals

ospital admissions are never fun, but for the older person, they are especially difficult, and even dangerous. And yet, for most people, hospital use becomes more frequent with age.

If you have ever been admitted to a hospital, you know it can be a stressful experience. If you are young and in good shape, you may be able to tolerate this insult to your personhood. But a frail older person with weakened coping defenses is a sitting duck. If you want to get really upset, rent the movie *The Hospital,* written by Paddy Chayefsky. It is an exaggeration, but not by much.

A person has to be pretty tough to survive the insults of a hospitalization. Just think of what happens. Your clothes are taken away by strangers. You are put in a strange environment with few recognizable signs to tell you if it is day or night. Your day is scheduled to fit the hospital's timetable, not your preferences or your needs. You may be required to stay in bed. Your sleep is disrupted constantly by noise and lights and repeated tests (checking "vital signs," etc.). You may be placed on powerful drugs. You will be subjected to complex procedures, procedures you may not understand. Not only that, but the air in hospitals is filled with antibiotic-resistant organisms. Looking at that long list, is it any wonder so many bad things can happen in well-intentioned hospitals?

It is ironic that the people who depend on hospitals the most are those with the least ability to cope with these stresses and threats. Professionals have spent a great deal of time thinking how to mitigate the threats of hospitals for children. Children's wards are often marvels of architectural and design creativity planned to reduce the stress of hospitalization. But much less thought has gone into designing geriatric wards, even though older people are the primary users of hospital care.

Hospitals are where we go for help, but especially for frail, older people, they can be dangerous places. Remember, one of the hallmarks of aging is loss of resilience. Older people don't adapt as easily to new surroundings as younger people. A hospital admission can be downright disastrous for an older person.

FROM HOSPITAL TO HOME

We rescued my mom from the hospital intensive care unit where she landed after walking into the hospital with a kidney infection. Although she had had kidney infections before, she was afraid this one was going to kill her, especially if it meant another night in the intensive care unit. So she chose to go home without any hope from her physician that she would live to see her next birthday a month away.

She lived alone in her own home, but two children lived nearby and neighbors and friends helped make living alone possible. The hospital bed in the small living room at first was intolerable. She thought how hard it was to die, how unfair that other people found an easier way to die. But she learned that it wasn't her time to go.

Neighbors and friends came to visit. She had always liked company and family caregivers didn't count for much. But each neighbor or friend brought relief from the tedium of bed rest.

Food at home trumped hospital food. At first my mom appeared to be losing her appetite for food just as my aunt did when she left hospital care for nursing home care. But at home, she could ask for whatever pleased her. Fried okra, fried potatoes, anything Southern-fried satisfied her taste. She began to eat.

—LYNDON DREW, CAREGIVING SON

Avoiding Hospital Mishaps

You can help avoid hospital mishaps by being aware of the risk factors and being vigilant. The list of possible calamities is long. Admission to a hospital may cause older people to become confused or agitated (see the Chapter Seven on delirium). It is also easy for older people to become overmedicated. Older patients recover from anesthesia more slowly than younger patients. Nighttime can be seriously disorienting, especially if an older patient leaves her bed to try to reach a bathroom. Older patients are especially prone to picking up hospital-acquired infections.

Even if everything goes technically right during a hospital stay, there is no guarantee that an older patient will have a comfortable stay. Older patients and hospital schedules mix like oil and water. Hospitals are often understaffed, and partly because of this, staff are under pressure to move quickly. This means it may be difficult for hospital staff to be patient—or to hold the patients' autonomous functioning as their number one priority. Instead, staff members are task-centered. It is faster to do something for an older person than to wait while they struggle to do it for themselves. This system can make older patients less functional, just at the time when they need to be working in the opposite direction. Hospitals neglect their rehabilitative duties in favor of efficiency, and increase dependency instead of encouraging self-sufficiency.

Patients with Vigilant Advocates Fare Best

Hospitals can be dangerous places even for relatively healthy people. Hospital safety and error reduction have become major concerns nationally. Older people are at special risk because of their underlying vulnerability. They need vigilant protectors. Hospitals are imposing structures and the power distribution is obvious. There are lots of "staff only" signs. Families are easily cowed by the efficient-looking, brusque staff in their operating room garb. Nonetheless, mistakes happen and those patients who have someone looking over the staff's shoulders generally fare best. We assume that the hospital staff know what medications the older patient was taking before her admission, but they may not. It is worth offering to review the list with the doctor or nurse in charge of the care.

Entering the Hospital

People do not go to the hospital when they are feeling fit as a fiddle (except to be fiddled with). People go to the hospital when they are sick or injured. The stress of hospitalization can make preexisting conditions worse. The hassles of treatment and the introduction of foreign substances like anesthetics and strong drugs can leave older patients dazed and confused. A person who comes in with mild confusion may become agitated. Agitation is treated with sedatives, which create more confusion. Get the picture of a vicious cycle?

When Hospitals Induce Delirium

Delirium, as discussed before in Chapter Seven, is an acute example of this disorientation. It should always be promptly and actively investigated. Even if an older patient doesn't develop delirium, hospitals can be disagreeable places. There are lights on at all hours and plenty of noise and activity around the clock. Addled brains are overstimulated and sleep is hard to come by. The intensive care unit (ICU) is even worse. It is called the intensive care unit because care is continuous. Obviously, some cases necessitate this kind of care, but with continuous care comes continuous interruptions.

Hospital Admissions Are More Common in
Institutional Living Patients

Long-term care institutions like nursing homes and assisted-living facilities are reluctant to assume any responsibility for illnesses or accidents. If a resident looks like she might be in trouble, institutions jump to call 911. You might think this trend would be more pronounced in nursing homes, but because assisted-living facilities have fewer trained staff, they are even more prone to call for an ambulance. Anytime an older person experiences an unanticipated problem, institutions summon the paramedics.

This strategy stems from several factors. First, institutions are concerned for the resident's welfare. Second, and this is a big one, institutions are concerned about their own welfare. Institutions work hard to protect themselves from litigation or regulatory reprimand. It's much easier to summon the emergency medical technicians—EMTs are essentially the paramedic rescue squad—than to take the risk of dealing with the problem themselves. It's also cheaper and less of a hassle. Long-term care institutions do not pay the costs of the ambulance ride and subsequent treatment. Medicare and the resident's family must pay for this care.

Once the EMTs Arrive

Once the EMTs arrive, the situation takes on a life of its own. EMTs follow strict protocols. First they make a cursory assessment and determine whether the patient is at any risk. With frail older people, it is a safe bet to say there will be risk. Then they transport the patient to the nearest emergency room.

This may not be the hospital the patient usually visits. It also might not be a hospital where the patient's physician has attending privileges. The hospital staff who treat the patient may know little or nothing about the patient's underlying problems. They may not even know what drugs they are taking. Most institutions do not take the time to send any of the resident's medical records to the hospital. This is a shame. On the rare occasions that a nursing home does send a nursing assistant and chart with the patient, these sources of information are extremely helpful—both for the hospital and the patient. But chances are this won't happen. When you are considering nursing homes and assisted-living facilities, ask about the facility's policies around calling EMTs and ask how they get information to the emergency room staff.

ER staff receive patients in the midst of chaos. They will be under pressure to act quickly. You have the right to know how crucial information about a resident's medical condition will be conveyed to ER staff. This information includes diagnoses and medications as well as a good history about the current critical situation. You should also find out how instructions are transmitted back to the facility. How do they ensure that treatment recommendations are implemented as intended?

Have a Hospital Admittance Backup Plan

Even if the nursing home has an organized system for dealing with ER visits, it is good to have a backup plan in place. You want to make sure that the hospital has all the information needed to best treat your loved one. Ideally, each resident of a nursing home or assisted-living facility should have a summary of their diagnoses and their medications. It is hard to find a handy way to keep an up-to-date record on a patient at all times. One good option is to use a MedicAlert bracelet. If you go this route, be sure to update the older person's MedicAlert any time her medical condition changes. The nursing home or assisted-living facility should be instructed to notify you immediately whenever your relative is sent to an ER. You will not be thrilled to be awakened but your presence is necessary.

Emergency Rooms

When is the last time you had a peaceful visit to the emergency room? My guess is your answer is *never*. Emergency rooms (ERs) are hectic environments, far from the best place to let a frail older person sit for several hours. As discussed in the last section, many institutions' first response to even minor problems is to send for the EMTs. Understandably, when these cases arrive at the ER, they do not get top priority.

ER personnel deal with urgent situations. A gunshot victim is going to be treated before a confused older person, obviously. As a result, the older person may wind up lying on a gurney (a stretcher on wheels) for many hours, virtually ignored. After EMTs deliver a patient to the hospital, their role in that patient's case ends. There is no one to stay with the patient. If the stimulation of the ambulance ride and the rapid change in scene did not do it, a long wait can cause a patient to become confused and agitated. Moreover, many older persons need to use the toilet frequently. What happens when an older person restrained to a gurney desperately needs to go to the bathroom? Nothing good. They may call for assistance, but these calls may go unheard or unheeded in the chaos of the ER. In a worst-case scenario, an older person may fall and injure herself while trying to free herself from the gurney.

My sister had to deal with frequent emergency room trips with my mother. She would get a call in the middle of the night to say my mother had fallen. The assisted-living facility would have already called the EMTs, who took Mom to the closest local hospital (which was not where she received her regular medical care). My sister would arrive to find my mother strapped to a gurney, disoriented and confused and crying out that she needed to go to the bathroom. There was usually no one around to help her. Invariably, my mother would eventually be seen, found to have no serious injuries, and sent back to the facility in much worse shape than she left it—agitated and confused. Our efforts to discuss the situation with the assisted-living staff were unsuccessful. Despite the potential harms of such unplanned trips, and even despite our offers to sign waivers of liability, we could not persuade them to resist their impulse to call 911 and set a chain of unfortunate events in motion.

Family Should Be Notified Immediately About Emergency Room Visits

In a perfect world, as soon as an older resident is transferred to the ER, their family would immediately be notified. In the real world, that notification may be delayed. If the nursing home cannot find contact numbers right away, that notification may even be forgotten. It may be inconvenient, but if you get a call that your older relative has been taken to the emergency room, you should try to get there as soon as possible. ER visits are one of the times when older people strongly need advocates. Yes, it is frustrating to sit—or more likely, to stand—with your elderly relative, waiting for your turn to be seen. But it can make a great deal of difference. You can help keep the patient calm, help her to use a bathroom, and make sure all her relevant medical information is made available. This is when you need your own lists of diagnoses and medications. (See Chapter Three.)

I am sure my sister did not enjoy standing with our mother who was on a gurney in the corridor of an emergency room as our mother moaned about how she needed to go to the bathroom. And I am just as sure that my sister was incredibly grateful that she was there with my mother, that my mother was not there alone.

Other Hospital Dangers for Older People

As I have said, hospitals can be dangerous places for all patients, but especially for older people. Older people are at a greater risk for all the typical dangers of a hospital. A serious concern is nosocomial infection. This term indicates an infection acquired in the hospital. Hospital-acquired infections, especially pneumonia, can be deadly, often because the bacteria that cause them are resistant to most antibiotics.

There are subtler risks as well. Imagine the series of misadventures that can befall an older person who is hospitalized. First off, being placed in unfamiliar surroundings is apt to create some confusion. Many older people, especially those with some degree of dementia, become confused around sundown. This "sundowning" syndrome is well recognized, although its etiology remains a mystery. Confusion can be exacerbated by poor vision and hearing, by being left alone, and if the older patient

has been given a sedative. Vision and hearing problems may be intensified if an older patient's hearing aid or glasses are misplaced, lost, or never
offered.

Now imagine waking up in a strange room in the middle of the night
and needing to go to the bathroom. If the older person has urinary
urgency—and most older people do—she may not be able to wait in bed
until help arrives. The dangers are still greater if she tries to climb over
bedrails. Many facilities are trying to lessen this danger by eliminating
bedrails and using sensors to monitor when patients get out of bed.

"Iatrogenic" literally means caused by treatment. Because the elderly
lose some of their ability to cope with stress, they are especially vulnerable to the adverse consequences of treatment. Their levels of resilience
are low to begin with, and when they get sick, those levels plummet
even lower. With one illness already attacking their defenses, it's easier
for another one to slip in as well.

Bed Rest

Hospitalized patients are often put on bed rest to facilitate the recovery process. But bed rest can have the opposite effect. Two groups of
people can get into serious trouble in bed: teenagers and the elderly. Not
only can prolonged bed rest exacerbate existing medical problems, it can
create new ones. If astronauts get deconditioned after a few weeks in zero
gravity in space, imagine what happens to a frail older person put to bed
whose muscles get no workout. They become weak. They have trouble
standing. They are prone to falls.

Prolonged bed rest can lead to clots forming in the veins of the legs.
When these clots break off and migrate to the lungs, it is called a pulmonary embolus, and it is life threatening. Pulmonary emboli can lead to
a collapse, circulatory instability, or sudden death. If prolonged bed rest
is a necessary step in your parent's treatment, take measures to prevent
pulmonary emboli. Special stockings designed to improve the return of
blood from the legs and to prevent its pooling there may be effective.

Blood thinners (anticoagulants) are another option. These measures may also be combined, and as always, be sure to talk to the doctor about your worries.

Resist Catheterization When Possible

What do you know about catheters? A catheter is a tube inserted through the urethra into the bladder to allow urine to drain out. Sounds pretty unpleasant, and it is. But in almost every hospital, the staff will enthusiastically promote the use of catheters. Catheterized patients are easier to manage. Think about it. No urinary accidents that can lead to skin breakdown, no trips to the toilet, plus an easy way to track urinary output. No wonder hospital staff push for catheterization. It takes real persistence to convince hospital staff to forgo catheters, and even more persistence to get them to remove a catheter once it has been inserted.

Risks of Catheterization

But resisting catheters is worth the effort. Excessive use of urinary catheters is one of the most common and one of the most serious iatrogenic problems. Catheterizing a patient breaks down the normal physical barriers that keep out urinary tract infections—a potentially deadly problem. If you have not heard enough, here is one more reason to avoid catheters. Even if an older person did not have incontinence troubles before catheterization, unfortunately, prolonged catheter use often causes patients to develop urinary incontinence. If it is too late to avoid the catheter altogether, one way to mitigate the incontinence problem is to clamp the catheter every two hours for twenty-four hours prior to removing it. Clamping the catheter means exactly that—one puts a clamp on the catheter for sustained periods of time to prevent urine from coming out of the bladder in order to prevent the bladder from becoming too contracted and unable to function properly once the catheter is removed. This can help to retone the bladder and prevent incontinence.

Gerontological Nurse Specialists Can Help You
in Your Battle over Catheterization

Despite all the problems catheters cause for patients, they do make nursing much easier. Because of this, they've become instinctive, a part of routine practice. You need to be prepared to go to battle over catheters. It can be hard to find allies. Physicians tend to be reluctant to be dragged into a fight over what they consider a nursing issue. They do not want to irk the nursing staff. Luckily for you, there are increasing numbers of gerontological nurse specialists at many hospitals. These specialists know better than to permit prolonged catheterization and they can speak the language of nursing. Essentially, these nurse specialists can be a godsend. You should seek them out.

Aspiration Pneumonia

Aspiration pneumonia is a greatly feared iatrogenic complication. Aspiration pneumonia occurs when the swallowing reflex is impaired. Typically, the entrance to the trachea (aka windpipe) is automatically covered when we swallow. This prevents food or liquids from entering the lungs. When that gag reflex fails to work, we literally inhale food and start choking and coughing. This is essentially the backup system; all that choking and coughing expels food that might otherwise have landed in the lungs. However, in some older people, especially those who have suffered a stroke, the coughing reflex may be suppressed or nonexistent. The loss of this reflex places them at great risk of inhaling some of the food they swallow. This foreign material can be the first step in developing pneumonia. If you are worried your loved one may be at risk for aspiration pneumonia, there is a simple way to test for it. Doctors can have the patient swallow barium (or some other radio-opaque substance), and watch the swallowing pattern under an X-ray. However, consider carefully the actions you put into play.

Pros and Cons of Preventive Measures for Pneumonia

Obviously, no one wants to get pneumonia. But it is hard to imagine anyone happily agreeing to the measures many nursing homes impose to prevent it. The preventive treatment for aspiration pneumonia can seriously damage an older patient's quality of life. Typically, patients will be put on a soft (aka pureed) diet and have all their liquids thickened. If your parent is put on one of these regimens, try tasting the thickened liquids. I have done it, and I will tell you, they are pretty disgusting. This is an instance where you should consider taking a knowledgeable risk. Ask yourself: Is reducing the risk of aspiration pneumonia worth taking the pleasure out of Mom's cup of evening tea? Take it from me, this question is never even considered by hospitals and nursing homes. They are simply focused on reducing their risk of liability. At least you should consider whether this treatment is worth it.

Effective Advocacy During Hospital Stays

Aside from the physical toll of hospitalization, hospital stays can cut back an older person's independence. Hospital admissions are times when an older person really needs support to continue to be self-sufficient. Unfortunately, hospitals often foster dependency instead.

First of all, hospitals concentrate resources on new admissions. Once a case has been diagnosed and treatment has been given, the patient becomes a lower priority. If an older person needs assistance with simple but vital tasks, like eating and going to the bathroom, she may get overlooked in the rush to get other patients to their tests and procedures. Additionally, overworked hospital staff can become impatient with slow-moving old folks. Nursing staff have heavy workloads, so it is not hard to understand why they may find it frustrating to wait and watch while an older patient feeds herself or walks to the bathroom. Helping an older person take care of herself is time-consuming.

I recall coming to visit my mother when she was hospitalized for an eye problem. It was Sunday. She was recovering from surgery. I was amazed and delighted to see how actively the nurses interacted with her (and she with them). I came back the next day to help with her discharge and could not get a nurse's attention despite active efforts. I had to feed my mother and take her to the bathroom. What had happened in those twenty-four hours? Weekends are a slow time in a hospital; not much is going on. Hence, the nurses have time to talk to patients. Once the pace picked up on Monday, my mother, who was ready for discharge, was a low priority in the scheme of things.

We can wish for more nursing staff, but it is better to do something; therefore, family advocates are especially crucial for older patients. But staff do not always welcome this kind of close attention, especially when it comes mainly in the form of demands for more care. Nevertheless, families must play the role of respectful advocates. You do not want to develop a contentious relationship with the staff, so you need to learn when to press an issue and when to let something slide. For example, it may be better for you to help your loved one eat while the food is still hot instead of taking time to track down a nurse and demand that someone be sent right away to help with eating.

Cultivating Empathy in Health Professionals

Good health care professional training programs try to increase students' empathy for patients by reversing the roles. For example, students wear Vaseline-smeared glasses, try to thread a needle with work gloves on, spend a day with popped popcorn in their shoes, or have cotton stuffed in their ears while being spoon-fed. Aggressive programs might give students enemas or an IV, or even have a nasogastric tube passed. A nasogastric tube is used for feeding those unable to feed themselves, or for administering some kinds of medications. Nasogastric tubes are pushed through the nose, past the throat, and down the esophagus into the stomach. Ouch! I am sure that students who go through this experience gain a new perspective on caring for older patients.

Even so, the hospital system is not designed to allow nurses to spend a lot of time on any one patient. Nurses have hectic schedules. Because of this, nurses may rush in to feed you or wheel you to the bathroom. These acts lead to debilitation. It is inadvertent, yes, but it is still harmful. Patients end up debilitated at the very time when they should be rehabilitated. Older patients need to be encouraged to do as much for themselves as possible, even if this takes a great deal of time and patience.

Transitions

The most vulnerable points in medical care are transitions from one situation to another. They involve the transfer of information that may not be done well. Sending patients to the ER or discharging them from the hospital or ER involves making plans and conveying information about what care has been given and what needs to be done in follow-up. Despite the vital importance of this task, it is often poorly done.

Leaving the Hospital

Leaving the hospital can be just as dangerous as entering it, even more so. Studies show that patients recently discharged from a hospital are at very high risk of problems, many of which lead to a re-admission. Even in the simplest cases of just going home, they may not be clear about what medications to take. Not infrequently, hospital physicians change a patient's medication regimen, either because her condition has changed or because the hospital staff did not fully comprehend the pre-admission regimen. Now the patient has two sets of medications—those they were taking before and the ones they are discharged with. What should she do with the medications she was taking just before admission? What should she look for as signs of problems as she recovers? What about diet and exercise? When should she see her regular doctor for a checkup? Does her regular doctor even know she was in the hospital, let alone what was done there?

Once a patient's immediate needs have been met, the hospital's thoughts turn quickly to discharge. Officially speaking, a hospital discharge must be ordered by a physician. But in practice, many physicians take little or no responsibility for planning the discharge. They simply delegate the whole matter to the hospital's discharge planning staff. The biggest role most physicians play in a discharge is signing the papers put under their noses. The discharge planner, who is usually a nurse or a social worker not previously involved with the case, is basically told, "This patient must be gone by five p.m. today." That becomes the prime directive.

There is a natural tendency to assume that the discharge planner is your friend and ally. After all, she is a professional; she works for the hospital that is there to help save your parent. She is *not* your friend! She is a hospital employee with a mission. And that mission is a prompt discharge. She may mislead in an effort to expedite. She may blame the urgency to discharge your parent on Medicare, but that is not true.

Why Hospitals Benefit from Shorter Stays for Medicare Patients

In most cases, this is how a hospital discharge goes down. First, the patient is approached by a discharge planner, who announces that the patient must leave the hospital within twenty-four hours. The discharge planner will suggest that Medicare will not pay for a continued stay in the hospital. They may even give the impression that any challenge to a "timely" discharge would constitute a breach of federal policy. This is not true! Medicare pays hospitals a fixed amount of money for each hospital stay, regardless of length. The actual amount Medicare pays is determined by the patient's diagnosis and a few other factors. Medicare simply states what it will pay, and recognizes that some patients will have shorter stays, and some will have longer stays.

Under this system, hospitals have a big incentive to keep stays as short as possible. Most hospitals are anxious to discharge patients as soon as their conditions permit. And remember, this is at their discretion, not Medicare's. In fact, Medicare beneficiaries have the right to challenge hospitals if they feel they are being pushed out too soon. If you suspect a premature release, you should inquire about formal appeals mechanisms. If you sense any reluctance from the hospital staff, it is worth consulting a lawyer, especially one who specializes in elder law issues. You can use a phone book or consult with an organization devoted to aging. A list of agencies on aging is provided in the appendix.

Don't Rush Decisions About Post-Discharge Plans

Making an informed decision about the best type and source of post-hospital care is a complex process that requires careful thought, good information, and enough time to work through the implications. Although hospitals, which are paid a fixed amount for each stay, would have you believe that patients must be discharged as quickly as possible, patients are entitled to a reasonable amount of time to make plans for their post-discharge care. Simply starting an appeals process can usually buy you enough time to make well-considered arrangements for your loved one. Long-term care decisions are hard, and you shouldn't be forced into making a hasty choice. Patients have legal rights. If you are facing pressure from the hospital, it is good to know what those rights are. Some key elements from the patient's bill of rights are summarized in Table 8.1. If you have more questions about patients' rights, the contact information for the Advisory Commission on Consumer Protection and Quality in the Health Care Industry and for the American Hospital Association (AHA) is provided in the appendix at the end of the book.

The Discharge Schedule

Two people will control the discharge schedule: you and the hospital discharge planner. Always bear in mind that discharge planners are employees of the hospital. They are not your friends or your advocates. Think of them the way you would a salesperson. They are selling you an early discharge. Basically, they are launch coordinators. Your discharge planner will probably learn about the upcoming hospital discharge on the

Table 8.1: The Patient's Bill of Rights

The following was adopted by the U.S. Advisory Commission on Consumer Protection and Quality in the Health Care Industry in 1998. Many health plans have adopted these principles.

Information Disclosure. You have the right to accurate and easily understood information about your health plan, health care professionals, and health care facilities. If you speak another language, have a physical or mental disability, or just don't understand something, assistance will be provided so you can make informed health care decisions.

Choice of Providers and Plans. You have the right to a choice of health care providers that is sufficient to provide you with access to appropriate high-quality health care.

Access to Emergency Services. If you have severe pain, an injury, or sudden illness that convinces you that your health is in serious jeopardy, you have the right to receive screening and stabilization emergency services whenever and wherever needed, without prior authorization or financial penalty.

Participation in Treatment Decisions. You have the right to know your treatment options and to participate in decisions about your care. Parents, guardians, family members, or other individuals that you designate can represent you if you cannot make your own decisions.

Respect and Nondiscrimination. You have a right to considerate, respectful, and nondiscriminatory care from your doctors, health plan representatives, and other health care providers.

Confidentiality of Health Information. You have the right to talk in confidence with health care providers and to have your health care information protected. You also have the right to review and copy your own medical record and request that your physician change your record if it is not accurate, relevant, or complete.

Complaints and Appeals. You have the right to a fair, fast, and objective review of any complaint you have against your health plan, doctors, hospitals, or other health care personnel. This includes complaints about waiting times, operating hours, the conduct of health care personnel, and the adequacy of health care facilities.

same day you do, which is typically the day of the discharge order. Their primary job is to streamline the discharge process. Do not automatically assume that the discharge planner has your loved one's interests closest to heart. Discharge planners must be efficient. In their eyes, the first train leaving the station is the best one to get the older patient on, even if it is not going where the patient wants.

Why Some Discharge Planners May Push for Nursing Home Care

Hospitals are dangerous places for older patients, so leaving quickly is not really a bad thing. The trick is to leave in an orderly, planned way. Arranging post-hospital care takes time. The more complex the arrangement, the longer it takes. A discharge coordinator's job is to empty beds. The longer it takes to arrange for post-hospital care, the more money the patient costs the hospital. Nursing home care usually comes as a fixed package. Home care, on the other hand, is arranged according to the client's needs. Home care takes time to organize and arrange. As you might guess, this encourages discharge planners to push nursing home care—even when other options also merit serious consideration. They may make it sound like any other choice is unreasonable and risky.

Making Deliberate Discharge Decisions

Making decisions about long-term care or rehabilitation requires careful planning and often involves hard choices. You cannot make informed choices without good information. Making a decision about anything requires (1) understanding the options, (2) weighing the risks, benefits, and costs associated with each option, and (3) clarifying primary goals or objectives. Much as we might like to be able to achieve everything, there are often tough choices to make. In the case of long-term care, clarifying goals can be difficult. Not everyone may agree on what is paramount. Some people may choose safety over freedom; others (often the older person) may opt for just the opposite. Families are usually active players (sometimes the dominant players). The more people involved in the decision, the more disagreement you can expect. You cannot make a rational decision when decision-makers are working in opposite directions. If the preferences seem irreconcilable, a mediator may be needed.

Steps in Decision-Making

Good decision-making around long-term care issues consists of two separate steps: (1) What type of care is most likely to achieve the paramount goals? See Table 8.2 for some issues to consider. (2) Who is best suited to provide such care? (See Table 8.3 for some issues to consider.) These two decision stages use different information, although concerns about cost and coverage may permeate both. The first emphasizes achieving goals. The second may be more about preferences. While the choice of a specific care provider may involve concerns about quality, other factors such as convenience, ambiance, and philosophy of care may also be salient issues. Or an older person may want to be in a facility that serves similar people.

Ideally these decisions should be made sequentially, but that is not always realistic. For example, your feelings about nursing homes may vary with the home in question. Some would simply be unacceptable. If there are no rooms in the one you want, that option may be off the table, at least temporarily. Or location may be a big issue. It may be better to choose a less desirable venue if such a location is closer to family and

Table 8.2: What Type of Care Will Yield the Best Outcomes

1.	What outcome are we trying to achieve?
2.	What risks are we willing to accept?
3.	What is the array of care options available?
4.	How does each option do in terms of achieving the desired outcomes and minimizing the risks?
5.	Which options are realistic? Where are there openings now?
6.	What are the costs involved in each option? Will third parties pay for some options but not others?
7.	Should we think about temporizing by taking a less desired option and getting on the waiting list for what we really want?

Table 8.3: Choosing a Provider for a Desired Option

1.	If a nursing home or assisted living, where is it located? Will relatives be more inclined to visit?
2.	If a home care agency, what is its capability? Does it staff with a full array of therapists? Does it have policies about weekend care. If your relative has special needs, for example, for a caregiver speaking a particular language, will the agency try to find such a resource?
3.	What do you know about the quality of these providers?
4.	What does it cost? Total cost? Net costs after third-party payers pick up their share?
5.	If it includes a residence, is it somewhere you would want to live? Who are the other residents? Will your relative have privacy?
6.	Does it have a philosophy compatible with yours? A religious or ethnic overlay?
7.	Are there policies that restrict the residents from doing what they want?

hence makes frequent visiting more feasible. Cost and coverage must be considered. If one type of care is covered and another is not, that may dramatically influence your priorities.

Comparing Nursing Homes, Rehabilitation Centers, and Home Health Care Options

If you want to make the best decision, you need to have all the information. When you are trying to decide on the best type of care for your loved one, you need to know the full range of the options that are available. It is easy to let a nursing home become your default option. Sending a patient from the hospital to the nursing home is easy and convenient. While other options might not be as simple to arrange, they're still well worth considering. The three basic care options are nursing homes, rehabilitation centers, and home health care. Nursing homes do not yield results on a level with rehabilitation centers, but home health care results are often just as good as those achieved through institutional rehabilitation. However, some problems cannot be readily managed at home. For patients who need continuing convalescence and rehabilitation, formal rehabilitation units can be a good way to go. Another option is to arrange for a combination of home care and outpatient rehabilitation. If a patient needs rehabilitative services, Medicare will pay for either inpatient or at-home rehabilitation. So a combination approach can provide a less expensive and more desirable alternative to institutional care.

Not Everyone Shares the Same Goals

Discharge planning can be complicated by disagreements within the family about the ultimate goals of care. Such crises often rekindle long-standing disagreements among siblings about who is favored or who has the most to say. These battles may require a referee. In some cases, a family therapist may be as necessary as a case manager.

Families Play a Major Role

Whatever option you choose, families usually play a big role in providing long-term care. You should decide early on whether the family has the physical, social, and emotional resources to be the primary providers of care. First you need to determine how much care is needed, and what kind. Table 8.4 shows a simple way to assess how much assistance your loved one needs, and in what areas of their life. When making this appraisal, be honest. If you have a case manager, ask her for her opinion.

How to Create a Care Plan

Some tasks, such as bathing, are needed once a day or less. Some have to be done regularly at fairly predictable times like meals and getting dressed and going to bed. Others can occur at less predictable times, like going to the bathroom. Once you've determined the care areas and the frequency with which care is needed, you need to plan out how that care will be provided. Try mapping out a typical week. Table 8.5 offers a way to think this through. You may be able to provide some of the care, but you will probably have to purchase help to fill in the gaps.

Table 8.4: Potential Care Needs

Activities of Daily Living (ADLs)

	Minimal or no human assistance	A little help	A lot of help/ dependent
Feeding			
Dressing			
Going to the toilet			
Transferring			
Bathing			
Mobility			

Instrumental Activities of Daily Living (IADLs)

	Minimal or no human assistance	A little help	A lot of help/ dependent
Cooking (if done previously)			
House cleaning (if done previously)			
Household chores			
Using telephone			
Managing money			
Shopping			
Laundry (if done previously)			
Taking medicines			

Incontinence

	Daily or more	Occasionally	None
Urinary			
Fecal			

Table 8.4 (continued)

Cognition-related problems

	Daily or more	Occasionally	None
Wandering (daytime)			
Wandering (nighttime)			

Assessing Your Ability to Provide Care

It is important for families to be honest when they appraise their abilities to provide informal care. It's not an easy undertaking. Giving care to a frail older person can take a heavy toll. Caregivers have been shown to have more physical and mental illness than those who do not give such care. Although families may feel a strong sense of obligation to give such care, making the commitment deserves serious consideration. One element of this decision-making should involve an honest self-assessment. Each potential caregiver should ask herself the questions in the Minnesota Family Self-Assessment in Chapter One and rate the results honestly.

Be Honest and Courageous When Considering and Weighing Risks

When you are making a serious decision, for instance, choosing a long-term care program, it is important to make sure you consider every part of the decision-making process. Maybe you have thought about your care recipient's needs, and the costs of different programs, and what kind of care you can provide yourself, but have you considered your feelings about risk? Especially if you're considering a nursing home, you need to give your willingness to take risks serious consideration.

Depending on the institution, the level of risks you are willing to take might be seriously curtailed. And you might have no choice in the matter. So before you commit, think about it. What level of risk are you willing to take on for yourself and those you love? Probably not a whole lot, right? But if you think about it, all of us take risks every day. Just driving

Table 8.5: A Simple Care Planning Tool

ADLs

	Expected frequency of task*	Who will do it
Feeding	Three times a day	
Dressing	Twice a day	
Going to the toilet	Several times a day	
Transferring	Twice a day	
Bathing	Every other day	
Mobility	Several times a day	
Managing incontinence		
Urinary		
Fecal	Several times a day	
Supervising	Constant	

IADLs

	Expected frequency of task	Who will do it
Cooking (if done previously)	Three times a day	
House cleaning (if done previously)	Once or twice a week	
Household chores	Once or twice a week	
Using telephone	Several times a day	
Managing money, paying bills	Once a week	
Shopping	Once or twice a week	
Laundry (if done previously)	Once a week	
Taking medicines	Several times a day	

*These are typical frequencies; you may need to adapt them.

to work, for instance, exposes you to a whole host of dangers. Nevertheless, when it comes to long-term care, many times people choose very restrictive options in the name of safety. Before you commit to a decision, talk to your loved one about it. Many older people are willing to take real risks if it means they can live more complete and satisfying lives. Do you really want to take that choice away from them?

As part of the process of your long-term care decision process, sit down with your parent and other family members and talk about risk. Compare your different levels of willingness to take caregiving risks. Talk about why each of you feels the way you do. Before you all talk, it might be helpful for each person to independently answer the questions in Table 8.6. Then you can compare everyone's answers. To gauge your risk-taking preferences, answer each question with "yes" or "no." There are no right answers; these questions are designed to provoke discussion. After you have independently answered the questions, compare the answers and use the discrepancies as the basis for a discussion of this important and generally neglected issue.

Discharge Advocacy and Case Managers

As with many other aspects of long-term care, when it comes to hospital discharges, you need to be an advocate for your loved one. In many cases, you may be well-advised to hire the services of a professional advocate. The point is that your loved one's best interests will not necessarily match up with the discharge planner's priorities. Hospital discharge decisions have serious ramifications. If you cannot devote the necessary considerable time and energy to handling the discharge process yourself, it may pay to hire a case manager. If there is family conflict, a case manager may be even more essential. Even if you do have the time and energy, you probably will not know the terrain. This is terra incognita for those who have never had to deal with these sorts of problems before. We do not know the language or all the options. We certainly do not have good information about the providers of each option. Case managers know how to work the long-term

Table 8.6: Estimating Risk Aversion Regarding the Care of Older Persons

		Yes	No
1.	Older people need special protections to keep them safe		
2.	Older people should be allowed to take risks just like everyone else		
3.	Older people need special treatment		
4.	It would be worth limiting an older person's freedom to keep them safe		
5.	I would feel terrible if something bad happened to an older person because I did not do enough to assure their safety		
6.	Everyone has the right to take risks as long as they know what they are getting into		
7.	I would prefer a safer environment for an older person even if it meant restricting the things they could do		
8.	Choice and control of one's life is very important for older people		
9.	Accidents can happen even if you take precautions		
10.	Fear of having an accident should not keep an older person from doing what they want		

care system to achieve the result that is best for your family. You and your loved one are their number one priority (more information is available in the Geriatric Case Managers section of Chapter Nine).

Make Sure You Receive and Retain Discharge Records

It is important to stay on top of all the elements of a hospital discharge. It can be a perilous process. Even with advance planning, discharges seem to occur in an atmosphere of chaos. Ideally, a patient should leave with a record of her stay and a clear set of instructions, including medications, for the next stage of recuperation. Unfortunately, this kind of discharge summary is

Table 8.7: Checklist: Discharge Data

Diagnoses treated (new diagnoses made, old diagnoses challenged, redefined)
Hospital course (major events, changes in medical status)
Procedures performed
Problems uncovered
Medications prescribed (final discharge set)
• New
• Old
• What was discontinued or changed?
• Reasons for discontinuing or changing prior medications
Activity level recommended and when normal activity can resume
Diet instructions
What observations about specific symptoms or conditions are needed
Follow-up appointments; which doctor will coordinate care henceforth
Plans for post-hospital care (e.g., home nursing visits, outpatient therapies)

not usually dictated until weeks after the discharge. Nonetheless, the patient should take with her at least a brief version of the discharge orders and the highlights of the stay. Families should know exactly what medications should be taken and when. Any changes to the preexisting medication regimen should be clearly noted. Table 8.7 lists the basic information families should take away from a discharge.

After the Hospital Discharge: Debilitation and Deconditioning

Older people do not bounce back easily from any misadventure. Each episode takes a toll. An older person may recover from an illness

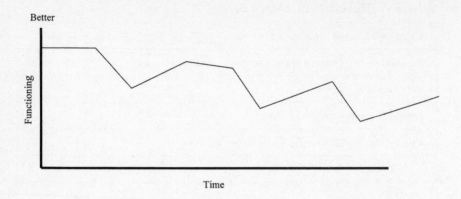

Figure 8.1: *The Pattern of Decline Often Encountered in Aging*

or a hospitalization, but often not fully. And after each incident, it takes longer and longer to recover. Basically, they never return to their normal level of health after a mishap. So each time an older person has a setback, it takes longer to recover and their ongoing level of health drops a little bit more. The gradual process through which an older person gradually loses his fitness is called debilitation. It is the opposite of rehabilitation. If you are put in a position where you are unable to use your muscles, those muscles will begin to lose function. As we've noted, even astronauts in peak condition will quickly show signs of deconditioning (such as loss of muscle and bone mass) when put into zero gravity in space. Most older people don't get deconditioned through trips to the moon, they just lose muscle function as a natural part of aging, but that pattern can be exacerbated when they are put on bed rest, for example. The overall pattern of debilitation in older people is shown in Figure 8.1.

Bed rest can act as a serious catalyst for the debilitation equation. When frail older people are confined to bed, they quickly become deconditioned. Older people begin with lower reserves, so it takes much less stress to push them into a debilitated condition. You should carefully consider the risks of confining an older person to bed. The idea that the best way to recover is to rest is usually wrong. Whenever possible, older patients should be encouraged to be physically and mentally active.

Prolonged bed rest after an illness or injury can have more negative consequences on an older person's health than the initial problem. Active rehabilitation, on the other hand, can help older people return to their pre-incident level of functioning and strength. In many cases, the super-vising clinical staff won't think about rehabilitation. So it is the family's job to press for it.

Rehabilitation and Recovery

Rehabilitation is not easy. After an illness or injury, a person feels tired and weak. Understandably, this can make him reluctant to com-plete the activities required for rehabilitation. It is hard to convince a person to walk when it's painful. But inactivity is the bane of aging. If someone takes responsibility for ensuring that the patient walks safely

Table 8.8: Questions for Rehabilitation Providers

Here are some questions to ask your rehabilitation providers to check up on the quality of their rehabilitation program:
• Who designed the rehabilitation program for this patient?
• How many times a day does the rehabilitation occur?
• How long does it last?
• Who does it? Physical therapists or aides?
• Where does it take place?
• How is progress assessed?
• Are there records of the daily treatments and the level of achievement each day?
• How is it reinforced (what happens outside of formal rehabilitation sessions)?
• Do nurses follow through on exercises that the physical therapists prescribe?

as frequently as possible, then the outcomes of rehabilitation in nursing homes and rehabilitation units are pretty equivalent; but that may be a big "if." Pain is a big part of the rehabilitation process. Pain medications are available and should be used. The best way to do so is to give painkillers before the pain becomes unbearable, and to take the lowest effective dosage. Table 8.8 offers some questions you should ask rehabilitation providers about their plans of care.

Family Members Can Help with Rehabilitation

As with many aspects of long-term care, family members can play a very helpful role in the rehabilitation process. Family members can actively advocate to ensure that older patients' pain is controlled and that drug interactions are minimized. Families may be hesitant to push professionals or other caregivers too hard. If you feel uncomfortable taking a firm advocatory stance, you might want to consider hiring a professional to guide and motivate care. Rehabilitation has a mixed reputation. Some worry that not all facilities that claim to provide rehabilitative services really do that. It is hard for caregivers to monitor what goes on outside the home, so rehabilitative providers may claim to be giving treatment when what they are actually doing would not match that definition.

Organizing Rehabilitation

It does not take long for older people to become debilitated and deconditioned. Even a short period of inactivity, such as a hospital stay, can have a negative impact on an older person's condition. After discharge, many older people need some form of rehabilitation to help regain the function and conditioning they lost during their hospital stay.

Rehabilitation programs differ according to condition. There are three basic types of rehabilitation therapy: physical, occupational, and speech. Physical therapy's goal is usually to restore limb function. They work with people to build up their muscle function, joint flexibility, and exercise tolerance. They help them walk. Occupational therapists help patients adapt to their disabilities so they can remain as independent as possible. Occupational therapy makes extensive use of assistive technology devices. These devices can help older people compensate for loss of function. They also make it safer for older people to function at maximum capacity in a real-world environment.

Companies have developed innovations to help make homes more user-friendly for persons with disabilities. One such example is the set of Lifease programs, which provides a system to assess a person's needs, abilities, and home, and then offers personalized suggestions that will improve the living environment. It includes a computerized assessment and a generated list of products that might help (www.lifease.com/lifease-home .html). It also offers BuildEase, which provides assistance in reconstruction (or initial construction) to make living space more disability friendly.

Obviously, speech therapists help with speech difficulties. They're also involved in minimizing swallowing problems. Sometimes, the line between physical and occupational therapy can seem a bit unclear. One way to think about it is that, in general, physical therapists address issues that involve the lower extremities and occupational therapists work on the upper extremities. All types of therapists work through assistants. Most of their time is spent assessing a patient's ability to function, designing a rehabilitative program, and then teaching others (assistants) to implement those programs. Ideally, the exercises the physical therapists teach are overseen outside of the formal rehabilitation period by floor nurses.

Post-Hospital Treatment Options Under Medicare

A patient's post-hospital treatments may include several types of care. Patients may be discharged from the hospital and sent to inpatient rehabilitation. From there, many patients return home. At this point, they will probably arrange for some kind of home health care. However, some patients do not return home after a stay in a rehabilitative facility. Instead, they are transferred to nursing homes. This nursing home care may or may not be covered by Medicare. Medicare does not pay for "custodial" long-term care. If Medicare determines that the patient needs to receive rehabilitative care, then the stay is paid for (within limits; Medicare covers the first twenty days and then imposes a steep copay for the next eighty days). A three-day acute hospital stay prior to rehabilitation is a minimum requirement for Medicare coverage.

Rehabilitation services covered under Medicare must be restorative and effective. Rehabilitation providers must document continuing improvement. For example, a person recovering from a repaired hip fracture may need active rehabilitation to regain muscle strength and walking ability. A stroke patient may need to visit a physical therapist to help with movement, an occupational therapist to learn how to perform basic tasks like eating with restricted movement, and a speech therapist to assist with talking and swallowing. This kind of rehabilitative therapy is covered, but physical therapy to maintain the current level of functioning and to prevent further decline is not. Even when therapy care is covered by Medicare, it is important to remember that after the first twenty days, a sizable copayment is required for nursing home patients. Nursing homes are paid by Medicare on the basis of a fixed daily rate determined by the patient's needs. Inpatient rehabilitation units are paid a fixed amount for their care package regardless of its length.

Choosing a Therapy Provider

After you have determined what kind of therapy is needed, the next step is to decide where your loved one is going to get that therapy. Many hospitals have specially designated and licensed rehabilitation units. Some hospitals even provide rehabilitative care as their primary line of business. These rehabilitative units often receive specially designated Medicare payments for the certified rehabilitation they provide. A patient will stay in one of these units until they meet their rehabilitation goals or fail to show improvement (aka plateau). Typically, this takes about two weeks. Just like hospitals, rehabilitation units are paid a fixed amount for each stay. So, once again, patients face pressure to leave as soon as possible.

Pros and Cons of Skilled Nursing Facilities

Depending on where you live, you may not be able to find a rehabilitative hospital or a hospital with a rehabilitation unit. In areas without such units (and in areas with such units too), rehabilitative care is provided through nursing homes. These homes are called skilled nursing facilities (SNFs), and they are Medicare-certified. Medicare also pays for rehabilitative stays in these SNFs. Unfortunately, research has shown that SNFs do not provide the same quality of treatment as formal rehabilitative units. The difference in treatment is especially pronounced for certain conditions—like strokes. Therefore, families of stroke victims should put extra effort into organizing treatment in a rehabilitation unit. If you must use a nursing home, find one with a real rehabilitation program. Ask specific questions about what services are provided, who provides the services, and how often. Are they employees of the home or contracted labor? What are their credentials? When you are checking out of rehabilitation, make sure the physician gives you a detailed program of what should be included in the rehabilitation regimen. This should include rehabilitation prescriptions, pain medications, and a plan for at-home care.

Home Health Care

Alternatively, some degree of rehabilitation may be delivered in a person's home as part of a program of home health care, which is also covered by Medicare. Here the care is much more intermittent. A physical therapist may evaluate the patient and oversee the rehabilitative regimen, but most of the actual care is provided by some type of assistant, usually a home health aide. Indeed, even in formal rehabilitation units, therapy assistants may play a central role in day-to-day care. The difference, however, is that nursing staff on the wards will, at least in theory, reinforce the lessons learned and practice the skills taught in formal therapy sessions. That reinforcement for home care falls to the family caregivers.

There are two types of home care, and they serve very different purposes. Home health care is provided through a certified home health agency (CHHA). This care typically follows a hospital discharge, and it may be covered by Medicare. This care lasts for a relatively brief time, usually less than six weeks. Home health care does not ordinarily provide care for the full day; it is used to provide additional, supplemental services. Long-term care at home is called home care. This care can be provided by the CHHAs, or by agencies providing more chronic care (these are typically licensed by the state). It is also possible to get long-term home care without going through an agency.

Home Health Care Assessments and Plans of Need

Most home health agencies are well equipped to quickly organize the initial assessment visit, but it may take a little longer to develop your care plan and arrange for regular help. For the assessment visit, the home health nurse will evaluate the patient. Based on this assessment of needs, the agency will develop a plan of care. The size of the Medicare payment is based on the timeline of this care plan, not the services included in it. Home health agencies are paid a fixed amount of money to provide up to sixty days of care. This means that once Medicare accepts the plan, the agency is operating on a fixed budget. The less service they provide, the more money they make. However, the care plan is essentially a contract. Unless the patient's condition changes, the agency must provide the services included in the plan. The problem then becomes what services get left out of the plan.

Home Health Agencies and Medicare Coverage

It may be unfair to suggest that most home health agencies gouge the system by cutting back on services. Most home health agencies are staffed by competent, concerned professionals. These people are anxious to meet the needs of their clients, but they are also pressed by what they see as the limits of the payment system. In fact, when Medicare switched to using the fixed price approach to pay home health agencies, there was a clear cutback on services provided. Often the agencies chalk their lack of service up to a Medicare requirement. But as you may remember from the section on hospitals, Medicare does not prohibit services; it simply does not offer an open-ended checkbook.

Screening and Overseeing Home Care

Welcoming someone into the home of a frail older person is an act of great trust. This caregiver is in a position to exploit and abuse. Fortunately, such situations are much rarer than you might fear. However, providing oversight for this kind of care can be difficult. Some people rely on agencies; others prefer to find an aide through word-of-mouth. They feel more comfortable hiring someone they know already or who comes recommended by others.

When you hire a home-care worker, you become dependent on that person. You rely on them to show up on time and you trust them to provide unsupervised care for your loved one. Home-care agencies screen applicants, but the screening process can be superficial. At a minimum, they should run a criminal background check, although some states have had scandals where former prison inmates have been hired as home-care workers. As those slip-ups show, there is no guarantee that the agencies will provide the level of oversight they should, especially if the demand for caregivers is high and the supply limited. Similarly, the agencies promise to take responsibility for finding a replacement for a no-show worker. But in truth, the agency may not deliver, and it can be trying to find a substitute quickly, which can turn into a frustrating situation.

Hiring Agency Workers Directly

As discussed earlier, despite the challenges agencies face, there is undeniably an added degree of security in working with an agency. And the agencies charge a hefty premium for that. Some people try to get the best of both worlds by hiring workers through an agency, and then contracting directly with the worker if they feel comfortable with them. This can be a win–win solution. The wages workers receive are substantially less than what you pay the agency. So you can often negotiate a price in the middle that saves money for you and puts more money in the worker's pocket. Obviously, this outcome is very unfortunate for the agency, as they lose both a client and a worker. Agencies try to avoid this by requiring clients and workers to contract their services for a set length of time, or demanding a fee if you hire one of their employees. However, if you have found an aide you want to work with, you can still hire him or her independently once this period of indentured servitude is paid off.

Live-in privately employed individuals prefer to work "off the books" without reporting income or paying taxes, not unlike the nanny market. You might rightfully worry about the illegal nature of these arrangements. Conversely, live-in workers who do report their incomes may also want and be legally entitled to Social Security payment and even Workmen's Compensation insurance. The bookkeeping tasks can be extensive. Like every other aspect of long-term care, this decision has to consider your parent's needs and what you can afford to provide, practically and otherwise. It also depends on your own comfort level with skirting the law.

If you are hiring workers by the hour, you need to weigh the benefits of using an agency. Home care agencies offer several advantages. They recruit and presumably vet the workers. They handle all the administrative tasks (i.e., Social Security, IRS). They presumably provide some level of supervision. They should supply backups if the aide does not show up. On the other hand, they add a considerable fee for all this service—sometimes almost doubling the hourly price. The aide may view herself as an employee of the agency first, and hence not be as responsive to your concerns as you would like. Very often families who find a worker through an agency ultimately try to hire that aide away from the agency to work for them directly. Typically the aide makes more and the family pays less. Agency contracts anticipate this maneuver and try to levy charges and provisions to offset this strategy.

Because it is hard to find aides, many families do turn to agencies. If you do end up using an agency, be sure you understand the terms of the contract. Many agencies demand a minimum amount of care per session. For example, each home visit must be at least for three or four hours (presumably to write off travel costs). Thus, if your relative needs just a little bit of help at several different times during the day (say getting in and out of bed), you may end up buying lot of unneeded (or at least less needed) care. Another strategy in recruitment is to ask friends and to ask the aides you like if they have friends who are interested in doing this sort of work.

Pros and Cons of New Organizations Providing Home-Care Services

The demand for home care keeps rising—and so do concerns about the costs. Because of this, new organizations are forming to help connect clients to suitable workers—all for a much smaller fee than the overhead charged by home-care agencies. One of the most popular is Home Instead, which claims that it places concerned, committed caregivers with older persons. However, it has been accused of high-pressure sales tactics.

Considerations for Overseeing Home Care

No matter how you choose to arrange home care, there are no easy or certain ways to be sure about what is going on when you are not there. It is important to appreciate that establishing home care requires a great deal of oversight on your part to be sure the caregivers show up on time and that they are doing a good job. Home care is not something that can be started and forgotten. It requires daily attention. You will have to train home caregivers to appreciate the preferences of your loved one. They will have to learn the routines involved in your preexisting caregiving routine. This takes time. Both the primary care providers and any backup workers who cover for time off must be thoroughly trained.

Time Off and Turnover

When planning for home help, it is crucial to consider the time and expense of time off for your primary home-care aide. You will need to arrange coverage. Even so, staff turnover can be a problem. Caregiver burnout can affect home-care aides as well. Some might have personal problems that force them to quit. Others might not provide satisfactory care and will need to be replaced. Every turnover involves a new episode of training.

Trust Issues and Home Care

And no matter how much training you provide, letting someone into your home to care for a frail older person is still an act of blatant trust. Not only can they rob the frail older person, they can abuse them virtually at will. And smaller concerns, such as failing to show up on time, can create ripples of disruption. Nursing homes eliminate that anxiety. There may still be concerns about theft and neglect in a nursing home, but it is a supervised environment. If you choose home care, and there are many good reasons for doing so, you will have to be vigilant about overseeing care until your home-care aide has truly earned your trust. Agencies presumably provide the oversight and do the screening, but their diligence may vary. It may not be possible to get a person to the home in a timely way if the key staff person does not show up. Monitor the care situation so you can quickly address any problems. Look for subtle clues, like the older person showing anxiety when you leave and the home-care worker comes.

Using Technology to Monitor Home Care

Technology can help you monitor a home-care situation when you're not around. One way to do this is through the use of so-called granny cams. These video cameras are installed in various locations in your loved one's home (especially bedrooms and bathrooms) and send a signal to a monitor set up in your own home. Some people view these cameras as an important safety measure, but others see them as an invasion of the older person's privacy. If you do choose to install granny cams, you should certainly talk to your older relative before doing so.

The list of technological aids goes on and on. It is amazing what is possible. For instance, it is now feasible to wire a home to track how active a person is, if they use the toilet, and even if they leave the stove on. Communication devices can send out daily reminders about taking medications, and you can even monitor when a pill container is opened. There are devices that can ask questions about a person's health status and determine when more attention is needed. Two-way video communication devices can make house calls from a fixed station. These devices cannot replace one-on-one personal care, but they may be able to provide assistance and improve supervision.

Other Creative Caregiving Solutions

Other assistive devices can relieve the pain of caregiving. Things like better lifts, bathtubs that allow a person to step in instead of having to climb in, and shelves of adjustable heights can make life easier for persons with physical limitations.

If you can, you should work hard to keep your older relative in her own home as long as possible. If you are willing and able to spend your own money (or your relative's), you'll have access to an even greater number of options than those available through governmental support public. If you are lucky enough to be in a situation where money is no constraint, you will probably be able to hire enough staff to take care of

One man's unique solution to the caregiving problem was to outsource the home care. According to a *Chicago Tribune* story, a man actually moved his parents to India and hired a team of home caregivers at a substantially lower price for the living situation and the care (Laurie Goering, "Man Turns to India for Cheap Care for Parents," *Chicago Tribune*, August 5, 2007). However, this solution might be a bit too extreme for most people.

a frail older person, at least for some period of time. If it is affordable for you, you can hire round-the-clock care. But for most people, money is a constraint, whether it is the older person's money or the family's.

Should Your Loved One Move In with You?

One option to think about, at least briefly, is whether a frail older parent might move in with you. Some families have made this option work. The best way, but certainly not the cheapest, is to build (or convert) some sort of semiautonomous living quarters for the parent. This arrangement allows for more privacy and a way to avoid always being in each other's way. Different families have worked out varying arrangements for meals. Some may be eaten together and some separately. This approach obviously requires planning and money. Because of the investment it should be considered very carefully.

More typically, arrangements are more makeshift. A bedroom is created, often by expropriating someone from their former haunts. This new arrangement means living in close quarters. For some families this has been the historical way of giving care and comes very naturally. For others, it can be a major disruption. Sometimes you have no choice and have to make the best of it, but many times a little honest introspection can prevent a great deal of resentment. As I have noted earlier, caregiving can bring great rewards as well as take a toll, but it rarely transforms a long-standing relationship pattern. Some families are not meant to be together and no amount of guilt can overcome those problems. Take an honest look at the past and make a clear-headed assessment of what seems reasonable, even if it means feeling like the ungrateful child. It may be better to scrape up money that is hard to come by than to take on a care burden that will not work. Table 8.9 suggests some things to consider about having a parent move in with you.

Nearby Independent Living Situations or Assisted Living: A Middle Ground

A middle ground may be to establish an independent living situation for your parent very nearby. Your parent could live in her own apartment,

Table 8.9: Questions to Consider Before Moving Mom or Dad into Your Home

Are you really going to be happy having your parent so near?
How well do you get along?
Will one party inevitably criticize the other?
Is your parent going to be happy depending on you for care?
Would they rather be cared for by a stranger?
Are you prepared to provide care?
What about your other commitments?
How will this arrangement affect the rest of the family?
How do they get along with the parent in question?
How will you handle meals?
How will you assure that all parties get some private time?

with whatever level of home care is needed. You could visit daily and handle whatever share of the care burden is feasible. We considered this option for my mother when she was about to leave rehabilitation. Because we had already moved her from her home in Florida to New York, it would have meant starting from scratch, finding and furnishing an apartment and hiring someone to be with her at least most of the time. Knowing how hard our mother could be on help, my sister quickly recognized that she would be spending huge amounts of time either placating the paid caregivers or recruiting and breaking in new ones. Given that she was a full-time teacher with heavy commitments, we determined that this arrangement was not feasible and opted for assisted living.

Chapter Eight—Points to Ponder

Hospitals are dangerous places for older patients.

Hospitals can induce dependence in older people.

Constant vigilance is necessary. Vigilance will reduce the likelihood of bad events occuring while an older person is in the hospital.

Emergency room visits are high-risk events.

Hospital discharge planners are not your friends. Their motives may, and most likely are, different from yours and your loved one's. Be wary.

Do not be bullied. Good discharge decision-making takes knowledge, resources, information, and time.

Rehabilitation is critical. Different types of rehabilitation can make a big difference in an older person's clinical course.

Nine

Send Help!

Good caregiving means recognizing that you *will* need help, and that the need for help often emerges over time as the stages of caregiving grow more intense. Every story of caregiving is unique, but most follow a similar trajectory of intensifying demands, needs, and stress. Failure to recognize and respond to the escalation of stress in caregiving can lead to a whole other set of problems. In one online support forum, one woman—I'll call her Mary—shared the story of her husband's experience of caregiving for her mother-in-law, who suffered dementia, mobility problems, and poor health. He was his mother's only surviving child.

For the first two years, Mary's husband worked hard every day at a stressful job but never took vacations because he left early each day to tend to his mother and take her to her appointments and such. He cooked, cleaned, shopped, managed errands and finances, and helped dress and undress her every morning and evening. He called her last thing each night and first thing each morning. On many occasions when his mother didn't pick up, he'd drive across town in the middle of the night to make sure she was okay and discover that the phone was off the hook. As his mother's only surviving child, this man was shouldering the entire caregiving burden alone, and he carried on this way until he was so exhausted he could barely see.

Mary helped as much as she could, but still the demands were staggering, and once in a while she and her husband would try to broach the topic of assisted living, but the elderly mother claimed she would die if they moved her. It wasn't until one day when the aging mother burned up the stove that the exhausted caregiving couple admitted she needed full-time care.

Looking back, Mary now recognizes four stages of care. In the first stage, she and her husband played the role of caregiver alone, running themselves ragged. In the second stage, they hired a woman to help in-home care. But Mary's mother-in-law hated being told what to do in her own house by an outsider. In the third stage, Mary's mother-in-law moved to a beautiful private assisted-living facility. After about a week of anger and resistance, she became extremely happy there. She enjoyed being well cared for and she had a great social life, which she hadn't had for years. She adored the activities director, and they formed a very tight bond that Mary initially thought was wonderful. She lived there for two years.

Mary's husband, though, was still feeling guilty over putting his mother in the facility, and he was spending most of his free time there, and his marriage of twenty-seven years began to suffer greatly under the strain. Eventually, Mary discovered that her husband was carrying on with the activities director at the facility. She faced the dilemma of either saving her marriage by moving her mother-in-law to a different facility, or leaving her there and further compromising the chances of reconciliation. What a choice.

Mary fought for her marriage. First she contacted the activities director and exposed the emotional affair to the facility's administration, and then she moved her mother-in-law to an Alzheimer's facility. By this time, the fourth stage, her mother-in-law's mental capacities had actually progressed past assisted-living capabilities and she had been asked to go to the dementia unit in any case. Mary's husband grew to accept his mother's condition and-in-law's tried to make amends for his inappropriate relationship with the activities director. Mary chose to forgive his emotional affair because of the awful stress he was under at the time. Though the stress around not "caring" for his mother full-time did not disappear, Mary's husband now realizes that he cannot do it all himself. Recently, the doctor ordered a CAT scan and kindly showed Mary and her husband how the size of the mother-in-law's brain had shrunk, the lobes had enlarged, and the veins and ventricles had atrophied or shrunk. Mary says that the damage of Alzheimer's and the stress of caregiving were the real villains of her mother-in-law's situation, not her husband. But in order to move forward, her husband had to learn to let go more and accept more help in caregiving.

Sometimes it seems as though you should not need to hire people to do what needs to be done. What is so complicated that you cannot manage it? But if you have learned anything from this book so far, I hope that by now you realize that in the world of long-term care, things are rarely as simple as they might appear. As my own mother's mental state deteriorated, she became disruptive. The assisted-living facility agreed to keep her on the condition that we hire an aide to stay with her at night. This seemed outrageous given the amount we were already paying, but it proved to be a no-win argument. The last thing we wanted was to have our mother become a pawn in a power struggle where she could become the victim. Moreover, her mental status improved dramatically when she got the individual attention her own aide provided. She loved it (at least most of the time). Having the aide also relieved my sister of the sense that she needed to be constantly on call. In the end, everyone was better off after the aide was hired.

Calling for Help and Behaviors That Tip the Scale

That situation with my mother is just one example of a moment when a caregiver might need to call for help. Sometimes finding help is critical to maintaining the current situation; sometimes it is about making a decision to make a real change, especially when that means transitioning your parent to another level of care or another setting. Deciding when to rely on paid assistance—or a greater amount of paid assistance—for a loved one can be gut-wrenching. It is a grave mistake to view recognizing needing help as a sign that you have failed as a caregiver. It is a central part of realistic ongoing appraisal of what is best for everyone. Your frail parent will not be helped by you exhausting yourself and your resources.

In some cases the need for more help may be precipitated by a crisis such as with my mother, but often there is no obvious sign of when to look for more help. The triggering event is usually a combination of changes in the older person's state and caregiver exhaustion. Certain behaviors can tip the scale. Wandering, inappropriate defecation, and physical abuse are common factors, but caregiver fatigue and exhaustion can be a factor and should not be ignored.

Caregiver Burnout Has Serious Consequences

At a certain point the physical, emotional, and social cost of taking care of an older person can be too great. Other family responsibilities are neglected, marriages suffer, and career demands present serious conflicts. Each caregiver must assess his or her own tipping point, but you should also listen to those who love you. Outsiders may see the signs of stress way before you do. You will likely turn a deaf ear, but at least try to hear what they are saying. Most often transitional decisions—the tipping points when we seek more help and greater amounts of intervention— cause caregivers to experience huge guilt. But just as often the caregiver is unaware of the toll being taken on herself and those around her. Sometimes it falls to others in the family to bring up the question.

Needing More Help May Require Institutionalization, but Not Always

Unfortunately, too often the question of seeking more help is seen as a question of whether or not to institutionalize, without recognizing that other available options can provide high-quality care. Older people usually want to stay in their own homes, or return to them after discharge from a hospital. And often that is the best alternative, but it may require heroic efforts. The stress on family members may not be worth the benefits to the older person.

Hired Hourly or Live-in Help

Many frail older persons cannot live alone, and hiring workers by the hour for around-the-clock care can be outrageously expensive, especially if you use an agency. A more affordable solution, which works sometimes, is to hire help from individually employed persons, including hiring live-in help. When you use an agency, a substantial proportion of the hourly fee goes to agency overhead. When you hire privately, the worker receives a bit more money and your hourly rate is substantially lower than it would be from an agency. There are very experienced people with up-to-date home health or nurse's aide credentials who prefer to work outside an agency umbrella, both because of the additional money and the greater freedom. Such individuals may be willing to perform tasks that only a nurse would be allowed to do if an agency were involved, such as clipping toenails or administering medications. Also, they may be willing to combine tasks such as cooking and housekeeping with personal care without the division of labor that agencies sometimes exact, and they may be willing to drive your relative in their car or his or her own car (though then you would be interested in the potential employee's driving record and, if using your relative's car or your car, you would need to be sure his or her insurance covers that employee as a driver). With private hires, the burden is on the family to do the screening and to check references; in theory, when you use an agency the reference checking and supervision are part of the agency overhead. It also is up to you to be sure that the employee arrives in time and performs the job well.

Live-in help is especially worth consideration if your relative needs a lot of general oversight and episodic help and if there is room in the household for an additional person. People looking for such a situation are usually will-ing to work for lower wages in exchange for room and board. Although they are expected to be available around the clock most of the time, they do need time off. A live-in employee needs both specific days off and some understanding about time to themselves during the time that they work.

Planning for this kind of care needs to include ways to provide reliable relief for the primary paid caregiver. For example, my father-in-law relied on privately paid live-in help who had regular duties for preparation of meals, laundry and housekeeping, assistance with showers, and escorting or driving him to places of his choosing. The schedule was rather regular but my father-in-law also sometimes needed quick help if, for example, he messed up the remote on his television and could not restore it because of his blindness, or he needed to answer the door or the telephone. Some-times people who previously worked in a nursing home on an eight-hour shift have trouble adapting to longer but more relaxed hours and respon-siveness to needs as they arise. The family caregiver may need to run inter-ference to make sure that a trusted live-in helper does have time off—to go to church, to pursue activities of interest, and to get away. The older person, who under the best arrangements becomes a friend to this paid helper, may become quite dependent, resist a backup helper, and fail to recognize that the job can be confining and tiring without adequate relief.

Look for Help Close to Home

The first place caregivers should consider turning to is their own fam-ily and friends network. Organizing that type of help requires time, and it cannot replace (nor should it replace) the paid help that provides personal care or nursing care. But these resources can play useful and important supportive roles. Obviously, not all family members are good candidates. Intrafamily relationships and histories are a big factor, but sometimes a crisis may change family dynamics for the better. You may not want to write off family members without at least giving them a chance to step up.

In the beginning of the caregiving journey, it is important to define who in the person's circle of friends and family wants to help, and what they are able and willing to do and for how long. Even out-of-town family members can provide assistance. These long-distance relatives may *want* to be part of the circle of support but feel unsure of what they can do to help.

Inevitably one primary caregiver is placed in or takes on the role of the "organizer." This person has to be able to recognize the needs of the older person and let him take the lead in voicing how and when he prefers help. But the organizer must also be honest about the situation and straightforward with the older person. Older people tend to minimize their lack of ability. The organizer–primary caregiver also has to be comfortable in asking people to help in very specific ways, being simultaneously persistent and diplomatic.

The first step is to realistically assess daily needs and capacity. This assessment will largely build off of ADL and IADL deficiencies. (See Tables 8.4 and 8.5.) The caregiver needs to identify and organize the list of "helpers" in the older person's *and* the family member's social network. This takes on the form of a matrix. For each potential helper you need contact information (names, addresses, phone numbers, and e-mail addresses), the types of help that each person is willing to provide, and any limitations that person places on her ability to help (e.g., tasks that she definitely does not want to perform, times of unavailability, etc.). Sometimes the caregiver's friends might also be willing to help, which extends the circle of support beyond the older person's social network.

Friends may be good sources of assistance with non-messy, non-heavy physical work like rides for errands, social activities, or some regularly scheduled, nonurgent medical appointments. Friends can help by bringing in a lunch and eating with the older person one day a week, or by offering other types of friendly visiting, such as acting as a reader or an exercise buddy. Sometimes friends can serve as "dinner cooks" who are willing to cook and freeze a dinner or two for use during the week. They might help with yard work or snow shoveling or shopping on behalf of the older person. Many of these things bring help and socialization—both of which weigh on an older person's mind. For example, a friend might go card shopping for the older person and pick up postage stamps so that she can send out birthday cards. Sometimes friends have special talents like shiatsu massage, healing touch, or Reiki.

Family members can tackle tasks like help with bill paying or taxes, filling out medical insurance forms, giving rides to medical appointments, seeing to light housekeeping help once a week, doing the laundry, tending to minor home repairs, or providing an occasional overnight stay or daily phone check-ins.

"CAN DO" FRIENDS

There are special "can do" friends who are even willing to be an overnight or weekend help occasionally for times when the family needs to take a break; e.g., if family have moved in temporarily for a few weeks after a hospital stay/ rehabilitation and are needing a short respite break. Mom had one friend in particular who would dive into laundry, meals, housekeeping, and visiting in a twenty-four-hour period, all the while interacting with Mom so that they had many good laughs.   —DEB PAONE, CAREGIVING DAUGHTER

INFORMAL SUPPORT

Even after paid help was being utilized, the family and friends network of support actually increased rather than decreased. I think the key was keeping them in the loop (mostly through e-mail updates I did), sending them thank-you notes, or giving a personal call, and (most important) my mom talked to many of them on a regular basis. Some of her friends also self-organized a lunch brigade for Mom with an appointed week for stopping in with a prepared lunch and visiting. I believe there were seven or eight ladies in that group. All told (though I haven't counted them all up) there were probably forty to forty-five people who helped out my mom at various times in the caregiving journey. Some were involved only once or twice, some regularly over the years.   —DEB PAONE, CAREGIVING DAUGHTER

Community Resources

In almost every community a number of agencies and programs can be tapped to provide varying levels of support and assistance. Table 9.1 lists a few of these resources.

Table 9.1: Home- and Community-Based Services that Can Be Tapped

Meals On Wheels
Driving/transportation programs
Chore services
Lifeline
Senior centers
Adult day care
Volunteer services programs
Faith-based parish nurse or other faith-based elder-focused ministries
Community resource centers
Local disease society (e.g., cancer, Alzheimer's, arthritis) that has specially trained volunteers
Nonprofit programs that focus on supporting the vulnerable in the community (usually through volunteers)

CHECKING ON CAREGIVERS

For every paid or volunteer program you tap into, ask about (1) background checks, (2) training/orientation, and (3) monitoring/supervision. The first time a volunteer or paid caregiver shows up at the older person's house, a family member should be there to check him or her out and be sure the person seems legit. Ask for identification, and take down the name and address and phone of the person and of the organization that "hosts" the volunteer or that manages the paid caregiver.   —DEB PAONE, CAREGIVING DAUGHTER

Handling Caregiving Crises

Caregiving crises come in all shapes and sizes. Veteran caregivers talk about the "crisis du jour"—that unexpected but inevitable crisis that requires immediate attention. Some crises are small, such as an incontinence accident or forgetting to pick up Mom's favorite kind of crackers at the grocery store. But others involve major decisions, decisions about turning points in a care trajectory. A caregiver can become ill herself, or even die. Or another family member's situation might change so that she needs care as well. A crisis on this level seriously shakes up a caregiving system. These are the times when you have no choice but to call for help.

In the midst of a crisis, however, you probably will not be thinking clearly. In long-term care, the best defense is a good offense. Life is full of surprises, and they are not all good ones. But if you map out a good long-term care plan, you can make sure that if something bad does happen, you already have an idea of how to respond.

Don't Wait for a Crisis to Seek Help

You do not have to wait for a major caregiving crisis to ask for help. Indeed, you absolutely should not wait. You should not try to take on complete responsibility for providing round-the-clock care for someone each and every day. Caregiving is draining. You need to take breaks. In the long run, this is the best way to keep you and your care recipient happy and healthy. Fortunately, there are many different care options that will let you take that much-needed time off. These types of care are collectively called respite care.

Respite Care

Respite care comes in many forms, and is meant to do just what the name implies: give the caregiver some respite or relief from the daily tasks. Respite care provides you with some rest and time to renew—or to do errands. It

RESPITE CARE

Respite care gives regular caregivers some time off and a much-needed break. Respite care is provided by:

- Home health care workers
- Adult day-care centers
- Short-term nursing home stays
- Assisted-living homes

Because respite care has a positive effect on sustaining caregivers, many Medicaid programs will cover it. Don't feel guilty about using respite care. It will reduce your stress, keep you healthier, and make you a better caregiver. Studies show that respite care helps caregivers keep their loved ones at home and out of institutions for longer periods of time.

does not matter what you use this time for—trips to the bank, pharmacy, or grocery store, or even a spa—what matters is that it is your time.

Many caregivers feel high levels of anxiety and guilt over leaving their loved one. Your anxiety over taking a break will probably escalate if your parent reacts poorly to a new caregiver. You might seize on your parent's resistance as a reason to call the whole thing off. But as I noted in the Separation Anxiety section of Chapter Four, this is the wrong way to react. No one can provide full-time care without taking any breaks. You won't be the exception to this rule. Do not try it. Eventually, your loved one will adjust to your absence. It might take time, but it is worth it, for both of you. Just as you may have felt that sending off your firstborn to school was abandoning her, you quickly come to realize that although you are probably the best caregiver available, others can manage in your stead.

There are two basic types of respite care: in-home care and out-of-home care. In-home care, obviously, is provided at home. This kind of care can be provided either by paid personnel or by other family members or friends. Out-of-home care is usually provided by adult day-care centers, but obviously for just one day at a time.

Adult Day Care

Adult day care may sound like a strange idea. But in practice, it can be a great thing for some caregivers and care recipients alike. Day care provides that crucial off-time for the caregiver, and it can be a fun, low-pressure, social experience for the care recipients if the older person enjoys socializing and if the clientele are compatible with the older person. Adult day care may work particularly well for a person with cognitive impairment—as long as the transportation and the hassle of getting the person ready are not too arduous. The day care experience is not for everyone. I never did well in kindergarten and doubt that I would ever tolerate day care in my dotage. Most adult day-care centers do not provide much in the way of care services aside from a chance to socialize. But some centers, called adult day health centers, also offer baths and physical therapy services. Occasionally doctors or nurse practitioners may even see patients on site.

Like child care, adult day care is often scheduled around the workday. The day-care programs expect primary caregivers to drop off their charges on the way to work, and to pick them up again in the late afternoon or early evening. Sometimes, the day-care programs' end times might require you to change your work routine. Some day-care centers send vans to pick up participants, but this may involve long trips to and from. Some older people enjoy such rides; others do not. Also, some caregivers have trouble getting their loved one up and dressed in time for the arrival of the day-care van.

Respite Care and Dementia

Older people with dementia can respond to care outside the home in unpredictable ways. Some patients become agitated when they leave familiar surroundings. For some caregivers, the stress of getting a confused person ready to travel can be greater than the relief obtained from the time off. Even so, other dementia patients do well in communal settings like day care. So if you are caring for someone with dementia, do not rule out out-of-home care.

Long-Term Respite Care

In some cases, nursing homes can be used to provide respite care. This kind of respite care is typically arranged to cover longer stretches of time. For example, families may temporarily place an older relative in a nursing home while they go on vacation. Families may also use these respite stays as tests to see how an older person adapts to living in a nursing home. In rural areas, small community hospitals may provide a similar service. If you need respite care but feel you can't afford it, you should seek community support. Your local Area Agency on Aging is a good place to start. You should be able to find respite services available at reduced costs—or even for free.

HOME CARE HELP

Both home health care or non-medical home care services help sick and disabled people live independently. Home health care includes health-related services such as medicine assistance, nursing service, and physical therapy. Non-medical home care services include housekeeping, cooking, and companionship.

Medicaid and some private insurance companies will cover the cost of limited home care. Coverage varies from state to state. Other times, you will have to pay out of pocket for these services. The cost of home care depends on what types of services are used. Non-medical workers like housekeepers are much less expensive than nurses or physical therapists. And some home-care agencies are cheaper than others.

Home Care as Respite Care

Home care can also be used as respite. Paid caregivers can come to the home to look after the frail older person, but it only works as respite care if the primary caregiver being relieved actually leaves the house, or at least does something other than tend to the needs or wants of the older person. It is not respite care if the regular caregiver hangs around to supervise the home-care worker.

Respite Home Care and Medicare/Medicaid

Unfortunately, this kind of respite care is not covered by Medicare or Medicaid. For some, paying for respite can be a financial burden they're unable to assume. In many communities, local agencies (like parish nursing services) can help identify volunteers who are willing to provide respite care for free. This can be a wonderful way to allow caregivers to take an afternoon off without the added guilt of paying for respite care.

Ways to Make Use of Respite Home Care

Home care can be used for the occasional afternoon off, or it can be used on a long-term basis. Long-term home care does not need to be overseen by a nurse, so it can be quite a bit cheaper than institutional care. However, organizing home care is more difficult than simply moving Mom or Dad into a nursing home.

Geriatric Care Managers

People need support when facing long-term care. The most objective onlooker would say that the long-term care system is complex and overwhelming. And besides that, becoming a caregiver is an emotional and stressful time. Having a dispassionate, knowledgeable advocate can make this difficult time easier. Hiring a case manager provides you with this advocate. Case managers (also called care managers) are skilled professionals who have in-depth knowledge about both the care system and the frustrations of dealing with it. Case managers are retained to work on the client's behalf but are not necessarily employed by the client per se.

Case Managers and Medicaid

Most often, case managers are government employees, sometimes working for the county or city, sometimes for the state. Their function is to assure the efficient operation of the Medicaid system (and perhaps whatever supplementary programs a state might operate). Much of their time is spent assessing potential applicants for Medicaid to determine eligibility, but they are also supposed to help families make more informed long-term care decisions.

They contract through these agencies to provide their services. These case managers work primarily with low-income clients who are enrolled in Medicaid. They assess their clients to determine their level of disability and their corresponding care needs. Then they construct a care plan. Depending on the generosity of the state's Medicaid program, this plan can include several alternative sources of care. Then the care plan is presented to the client and their family. Some negotiations are possible at this stage. Following this meeting, the case manager is charged with implementing the plan. They contact agencies that provide the approved services and authorize an agreed-upon amount of care. The care manager then monitors the situation to be sure that the services are provided and that they are of adequate quality.

Case Managers and Conflicts of Interest

As I have said earlier, most long-term care professionals have their own concerns. It is not always easy to distinguish case managers who work for agencies from those who work for clients. Discharge planners, for example, are employed by hospitals and nursing homes. They serve a similar purpose as care managers, but their primary responsibility is to see that their employing organization's agendas are met. I talked earlier about the dangers of relying too heavily on hospital discharge planners and physicians. These professionals may mean well, but they may also have conflicts of interest, and you are not their only client (or even their major client).

Many professionals have only limited knowledge about the range of long-term care options and the intricacies of treating frail older patients. They may choose to simply rely on their own personal experience. Some physicians have attending privileges at a limited number of facilities, which means those are the facilities they are inclined to recommend. The advantage to this arrangement is a greater potential for continuity of care, but the disadvantage is that you are cutting off options without even knowing it.

In some cases, a physician may have direct financial interests in a nursing home. It might be a difficult topic to broach, but it's wise to ask your doctor if she has a financial interest in the home they've recommended, and if there are other homes—perhaps ones where your doctor also has practice privileges—that are as good or better.

Private Case Managers

There is a burgeoning industry of private case managers, who work directly for clients. A private case manager works on behalf of the older person—and perhaps their family. These case managers are the only long-term care professionals who truly work for the patient. A private case manager is an advocate. A case manager's job is to help the family members make the best decisions they can and to implement those decisions or assist the family in doing so. This means giving the family good advice about the choices available to them, along with information about the risks, costs, and benefits attached to each choice. A case manager can work with the family to identify what aspects of care are the most important and which outcomes they hope to maximize.

Private Case Managers and Conflicts of Interest

Just because you have hired the case manager, however, does not mean you are the only one paying them. Would you fully trust an investment counselor who works on commission or who is paid by certain companies for purchases of their stocks? I hope not. These same conflicts of interest exist in the long-term care world. You need to identify any potential conflicts of interest. You should not rely on advice from someone who is an employee of a nursing home or a hospital, or who receives commissions or kickbacks. It may be hard to find out about such incentive payments. The only way to know is to ask. Especially when you're hiring a case manager, be sure to ask directly about the candidate case manager's background and any connections to care providers and facilities.

The Older Person Should Be the Client

Case managers tend to view themselves as working for the person who pays them, but that is not necessarily the best policy. It is very important to make it clear from the beginning that the client should be the older person, and to repeatedly reinforce the idea if necessary. The goal is to avoid bypassing the care receiver. The older client should be at the center of any discussions and decisions. One principle to always remember is that older people, even those with dementia, should never be discussed in the third person in their presence.

It is important to determine upfront for whom the case managers are advocating. Many case managers and families believe that the case manager should work for the person hiring them. Other parties argue that case managers should consider the care receiver as their primary client regardless of who does the hiring. A third party may hire a lawyer on a client's behalf, but the lawyer is still responsible to the client, not to the hiring party.

Case managers are usually hired by family members. However, just like lawyers, their real concern should be the older person—their client.

Families often feel protective and may infantilize the care recipient by taking over decision-making roles. This means the reporting responsibility for a case manager can become complicated. Make sure to clearly establish this level of accountability.

When we hired a case manager to help with our mother's care when she was living on her own, it took a long time to convince the case manager that our mother was the primary client, not us. His job was to address her needs and involve her in decisions, not to please us (although he could hardly afford to alienate us).

Considerations in Hiring a Case Manager

You should put as much time and care into hiring a case manager as you would with a lawyer. Find out about their training and experience. Ask for references. Check with the national certifying organizations—the Case Management Society of America, the Center for Case Management, Inc., and the National Association of Social Workers (contact information is provided in the appendix). But in each instance, remember that it's unclear just what such organizations' credentialing really means; a lot of these certifications may simply involve paying dues. Try to find a care manager who has worked in the field of aging for a while. Ideally, your care manager should have a background in social work or gerontology.

Resources for Locating Case Managers

There is a national association for case managers (Case Management Society of America), and several case management services are listed on the National Association of Professional Geriatric Care Managers website (contact information for these and the following organizations is listed in the appendix). Unfortunately, just as with lawyers and other types of advocates, there is no easy way to measure how well a given case manager or a case management company performs. There is no state certifying body and no records of their performance. Yes, there is a national certification system, but it is run as a commercial operation. Certification only guarantees that the case manager paid for a course of study and a certifying examination.

One way to find a case manager locally is to look for a nearby hospital that has a geriatric program. Call the hospital and ask for a referral to a reliable case manager. Alternatively, contact your local Area Agency on Aging (AAA). These Area Agencies are supported by a federally funded program designed to help older people and their families. Telephoning 800-510-2020 will automatically connect you with the nearest AAA, but depending on where you live, this may not be the agency nearest to your care recipient. The National Administration on Aging also has a Web-based Eldercare Locator you can use to find a case manager. It might not be easy to find a case manager, but can be terribly important for the well-being of the older person, especially during a crisis.

Given the lack of well-developed criteria and certification, probably the best way (but certainly not the easiest way) is to ask a friend who has used one, if you can find such a person. At a minimum, ask for references (and check them) before hiring a case manager.

What to Expect from Case Managers

As an advocate, the case manager is expected to work the system on her client's behalf. She is not there to protect society's interests. She may suggest somewhat sneaky ways to make older people eligible for public programs. Most case managers are not estate planners, so they may need to refer the family to these planners. Estate planners know more about the ins and outs of divestiture. They can help families shuffle assets around to establish eligibility for Medicaid. However, many older people and their families are reluctant to find ways to take advantage of the system unless their situation is desperate.

Good case managers should know which agencies provide the best care. They should work with those agencies to ensure that the needed care is provided consistently and provided well. Case managers have two important advantages in ensuring this care: First, they are more knowledgeable and experienced. Second, they can deal with the agencies dispassionately; they do not bring a lot of emotional baggage to the table. Case managers should know what to expect from service providers and how to assure that the client is adequately served.

Long-Distance Case Management

Another difficulty with the accountability structure is that the caregiver, the older person, and the case manager may not all live in the same place. There is a growing trend for local case managers to be hired to act as on-site surrogates for children living at a distance who cannot be there to manage care in person all the time. In theory, these case managers can keep an eye on things and intervene when necessary. In practice, the case manager is expected to function as an extension of the adult child. Obviously, this assignment can lead them to consider the adult child as their primary client. These case managers are prone to defer to the children's wishes rather than the older person's. This interferes with the older person's autonomy and compromises their privacy. Especially when organizing care from a distance, it can be hard to avoid this situation. Once again, emphasize that the case manager works for the older client, not for you. Try to prioritize your older relative's wishes above your own. The fewer disagreements between the two of you, the fewer opportunities for an accountability snarl.

Chapter Nine—Points to Ponder

You cannot do it all yourself. In order to buffer themselves against the demands of giving care, many caregivers convince themselves that they are indispensable, that no one else can give the needed care quite as well as they can. That may be true, but you will not be able to sustain the task if you do not accept help. You should feel free to ask for help. Set up a family meeting and determine what other family members are willing to do to help out.

Take advantage of respite care. You need to get away and take care of other business, lest caregiving become an all-absorbing activity and ultimately take an even heavier toll.

Be willing to buy help. Even if you provide most of the care, it may be good to hire someone to spell you or just to share the burden.

Finding good home-care aides is hard. You may need to start with an agency.

Day care is good for some older people but not for all.

Case managers can be a big help, but you need clear ground rules.

Ten

Moving Time

An older person will almost always want to stay in his or her own home. And in many cases, staying at home truly is the best option. But sometimes, it may not be possible. As noted in Chapter Nine, organizing at-home care takes a whole lot of time and sometimes a whole lot of money. In-home care may cost less than a nursing home stay, but the third-party coverage is often less generous.

MOVING ONE STEP AT A TIME

My eighty-seven-year-old dad and I were at the doctor's office for a medical exam for Dad. The question I needed to ask was, "How do you decide when it is no longer safe for Dad to live at home with Rose (my fifty-year-old mentally challenged sister)?" Our family knew that the nine hundred people in the town were talking about Dad's situation, and we were concerned. The doctor said, "Something will happen and you will know that it is time."

We had caregivers who came to the house every day. They cleaned and cooked for Dad and my sister. One of the caregivers had the ability to understand Dad. Every morning when Dad got up he said, "I'm not sure that I will make it through the day." Joyce would respond, "Let me get you some breakfast, Ralph, and then let's see how you feel." Needless to say, Dad was better after breakfast.

(story continued)

The other caregiver, unfortunately, had a tendency to respond to Dad's morning grousing by calling 911! I convinced her to call me before she called 911. Later on, Dad started going to sleep after the caregiver left in the afternoon and would get up around midnight to go to the bank. My sister would call me. I would talk to Dad on the phone for a while and then say, "You know, Dad, it's bedtime now. Put your pajamas on and go to bed now." After this happened a few times, we decided to have another caregiver come to the house in the later afternoon to keep Dad up until it was time to go to bed.

This worked for a while, but then it quit working on the days that she did not come. By now, the calls from my sister were coming three times a week and Rose was losing weight from the stress of it all. One day another call came from Linda, one of Dad's caregivers. "Your dad says that he isn't feeling well this morning," she said. I told her to put Dad on the phone, and I said to him, "Dad, you don't feel well this morning. Do you think that it is time for you to go live at a place with nurses to take care of you every day?" "I think so," he replied.

I made the arrangements for him to enter a home in northern Iowa. Several days later, my sister–in-law, who was a nurse in a nursing home, and I picked up Dad and took him to the nursing home. We knew that it was the right time. Dad lived there for four years.

—JOANN HOWITZ, CAREGIVER AND PHYSICAL THERAPIST

Long-term care decisions are usually made because an influential party (the family caregiver, or a professional who may be a doctor or more likely the administrator of a facility) has determined that a certain option is no longer viable. When discussing long-term care options, it is better to be honest and not raise unrealistic expectations. Discussions will be more productive if the options are limited to what the pertinent parties consider doable. However, you should try to be open-minded. Do not foreclose options too quickly. I am often asked for help in finding placements for people by family members who have defined the question in terms of an answer. They start out asking me to recommend a good nursing home and are surprised when my first response is, "Why do you think you need a nursing home?" They have, in effect, closed off other, perhaps more suitable options at the outset. My job then is to widen their horizons. In some cases, strength of will can out-trump reason. An older person may truly prefer to survive in conditions you see as unworkable rather than give up their familiar surroundings.

When you hit a serious mile marker decision in your long-term care journey—for instance, moving an older person out of their home—you want to approach that decision very carefully and very systematically. Long-term care decisions carry heavy emotional weight, but you need to try to make rational choices nonetheless. Table 10.1 provides a good structure for choosing the best type of long-term care for your loved one, and also for choosing a care provider.

Know What Matters Most to Your Loved One

The art of negotiating (and decision-making) lies in being clear about what is most important. That is the thing you do not want to yield on. It is crucial to identify what matters most to the older person in question (and to you). Some people place great stock in protecting their independence, both physical and social. However, there are times when, whether we want to or not, we have to follow arbitrary routines. Sometimes, we have to accept that the means justify the ends. When you enter a hospital, for example, you may have to endure indignities. But you are willing to do so, because you are hoping to receive a great benefit at the end—improved health. Some people have no problem with following an institution's preferred routines, if that allows them to get the needed care. Other people rebel against the system. Enduring indignities shouldn't be the price we pay for health, but sometimes it is. Ideally, we should not have to choose between our health and our dignity. But the long-term care world is full of compromises.

That does not mean an older person has to shift from living on her own to living in a nursing home. For many, there are several steps in between. When you decide it is time to move, do not automatically

Table 10.1: Things to Consider for Making Good Choices

Nature of decision	Basic questions	Resources
What kind of LTC is most appropriate?	Which type of care will maximize the outcomes that are most important? Nursing home Rehabilitation unit Home health care Home care Assisted living Day care What outcomes do we want to maximize? Autonomy, independence Safety Comfort Quality of life What types of care are covered by available insurance (including government support—Medicare, Medicaid, Veterans Administration)?	A case manager (or care manager) may be crucial in helping you work through what outcomes are most important. She may also have access to actual data about what types of care can best achieve the goals.
Who should provide the LTC?	What is the quality of the care provided? How convenient is the location? What amenities are provided? How do the policies correlate with my preferences? How often in the past several years has the leadership (especially the administrator and director of nursing) and the other staff turned over? Do they pay benefits to staff?	You will probably need to ask the specific potential providers these questions. The Department of Health in every state has some information on providers of some forms of LTC. Some states post information on providers on their websites. Medicare's Nursing Home Compare website provides some data on quality for all nursing homes. Ask for the most recent state survey report.

default to a nursing home. In many cases, it is feasible to give good care in a setting that allows older people to live essentially as they please. The catch is, it may take some looking to find those places.

Choosing the Best Long-Term Care Program

If you have decided that informal care will not meet your care needs, then it is time to explore formal care options. Table 10.2 summarizes the major forms of long-term care.

Table 10.2: Types of Long-Term Care

LTC type	Description
Nursing facility	All nursing homes are certified to provide care at one or more levels. Many nursing homes are certified to provide post-hospital care under Medicare—these are referred to as skilled nursing facilities. Long-term care nursing facilities are certified to provide long-term care funded either privately or through Medicaid. Nursing homes must provide at least minimal levels of nursing staff and have an infrastructure capable of overseeing the care of frail persons.
Home health care	Medicare certified care that's operated under the jurisdiction of registered nurses. Other core staff include physical, occupational, and speech therapists, and social workers. Most care is provided by home health aides. Patients usually require some form of active nursing care and supervision. Most of the care is directed at recovery after a hospitalization.
Home care/ personal care	Services provided to support a frail person who needs assistance in meeting various ADL or IADL care. Nurses may supervise, but most care is provided by personal-care aides or homemakers. In many cases people may purchase this care directly, contracting with individual aides. Home care, as distinct from home health care, is not covered by Medicare but is covered by Medicaid.
Rehabilitation units	Specifically licensed facilities that can provide active rehabilitation. These are usually distinct units of a hospital (not all hospitals), but some are freestanding. Care must be under the direction of a specialist physician, called a physiatrist. Most of the care is given by nurses and physical and occupational therapists, although aides may carry out most routines. Occupational therapists and speech therapists may be actively involved.

Table 10.2 (continued)

Assisted living	Institutional care where residents live in self-contained units that include living quarters, a private bathroom, and some modest cooking and food storage facilities. Assisted-living residents are first and foremost tenants. They may use a common dining room and participate in various organized activities, but they control their routines and should be able to decide who enters their living space. The facility provides some basic support services under various payment arrangements, Assisted-living facilities may serve a wide variety of clients, but usually they serve a less disabled clientele than nursing homes. Staffing varies quite extensively, in part depending on the populations they seek to serve. In general, assisted living provides less nursing care and less active involvement in treatment. They may refuse to care for a person whose condition deteriorates past the point where they feel comfortable providing the necessary type and amount of care. Most assisted living is paid for privately. Medicaid coverage of assisted living varies by state but is generally not as good as what is available privately.
Day care or adult day health center	Care provided in centralized facilities for various periods of the day. The goal of this care is twofold—first, to provide socialization for older persons otherwise confined to their homes, and second, to provide relief (respite) for family caregivers. Some day-care programs provide organized activities and may also provide services like assistance with ADLs and even bathing. Some day-care sites also have medical or nursing services on the premises (often referred to as adult day health care in contrast to social adult day care).
Hospice/palliative care	Hospice care is intended for those who've reached the expected terminal phase of life. The typical prognosis is less than six months. Hospice care is a benefit under Medicare. In effect, a person choosing that option waives her rights to traditional care and enters a program designed to make the end of life as peaceful and pleasant as possible. Most hospice care is given at home. Hospice goals address the alleviation of uncomfortable symptoms, like pain, nausea, constipation, and itching, and provide the support needed to face death.
Palliative Care	A related service is called palliative care. It differs from hospice care in not being an explicit Medicare benefit. It uses many of the same approaches but does not imply a decision to forgo active treatment. Thus, it can address the unpleasant effects of dying in a more clinical context.

Table 10.2 (continued)

Continuing Care Retirement Communities[14]	These are designed as one-stop shops. In theory a person can move in as a healthy retiree and receive needed care in increments as their need increase. On a single campus one will find apartments (even town houses), home care, assisted living, and a nursing home. Payment as disability increases may reflect the additional needed services or it may be more of an insurance arrangement. Some CCRCs have their own medical staff.

There are some important differences in the coverage for hospice and palliative care, as summarized in Table 10.3.

Table 10.3: Coverage Differences Between Hospice and Palliative Care

Question	Hospice Care	Palliative Care
Does Medicare pay?	Medicare pays all charges related to hospice	Some treatments and medications may be covered
Does Medicaid pay?	In forty-seven states, Medicaid pays all charges related to hospice	Some treatments and medications may be covered
Does private insurance pay?	Most insurance plans have a hospice benefit	Some treatments and medications may be covered
Is this a package deal?	Medicare and Medicaid hospice benefits are package deals	No, there is no "palliative care package"; the services are flexible and based on the patient's needs
How long can I receive care?	As long as you meet the hospice's criteria of an illness with a life expectancy of months, not years	This will depend upon your care needs, and the coverage you have through Medicare, Medicaid, or private insurance

Source: Janet Gibson, *The Complete Guide for Senior Care* (Minneapolis: WiseLife Press, 2007).

---

14. CCRCs are not really a specific service but a way of providing a range of services.

Continuing Care Retirement Communities

If none of the basic options sounds right for your parent, you might want to see if there are any Continuing Care Retirement Communities (CCRCs) in your area. These programs try to provide a variety of different service options at the same location. CCRCs may be run for profit or they may be sponsored by non-profit organizations, usually organizations with religious affiliations. The financial arrangements also vary by institution.

Typically, you pay a (sometimes refundable) deposit upon admission to a CCRC. After that point, residents pay a monthly fee for an apartment and some minimal services. For instance, one meal a day is included in many packages. After that basic level, extra services come with extra fees. Most residents enter CCRCs in a pretty independent condition. Initially, it serves as a retirement home. As a resident's care needs increase, it may become necessary for them to move into a more supportive environment. They can transition from self-sufficient living to assisted living and eventually into the skilled nursing units without leaving the campus. Each move to a higher care unit comes with a higher price tag.

This all-in-one approach minimizes dislocation, which is very appealing to many people. Hopefully, friends made on site will maintain their relationships as their care needs change. Some people see this as a way to "age in place," expecting that they can remain in their apartments and simply receive more services. Experience suggests that this does not usually happen. There are pressures from all sides to move up to higher levels of care. The administration wants to keep its high-care beds full and neighbors may not welcome frail people in their midst. The actual financial arrangements vary. In most instances, the costs increase with each step, but some CCRCs provide within the fee structure a form of long-term care insurance, by which you may pay a large entry fee that, in effect, provides coverage for higher care needs. It is important to understand precisely what is in the contract you are signing. The contracts can be very complex. Professional assistance and advice should be sought.

Mixed Experiences with Continuing Care Retirement Communities

The experience with CCRCs is mixed. Some deliver what they promise. Others run into financial difficulties, or don't have a space available in the assisted living or nursing home unit when it's needed. Arranging for home care, where services are brought into the person's apartments, can be difficult. There can also be conflict among the residents. Relatively healthy residents do not always deal well with the presence of frailer individuals. They claim that they came to the CCRC to be with other healthy people, and object to any hints of a nursing home environment. It will be interesting to see how these hiccups resolve as the CCRC system itself grows older.

Program of All-Inclusive Care for the Elderly (PACE)

One of the most exciting developments in the long-term care world is the PACE program. The PACE program proves that it is possible to receive good medical and long-term care without resorting to entering a nursing home. The program began in San Francisco and has spread across the country. Unfortunately, the PACE program is available to only a very small group of people. It serves only those who are eligible for both Medicare and Medicaid and who are eligible for nursing home care, but who are still living in the community.

PACE is designed to keep participants out of nursing homes and hospitals by providing highly integrated care. PACE care is mainly provided through adult day health centers. These centers employ physicians who believe in the PACE model. The program emphasizes teamwork and egalitarianism; it actively encourages all the employees (from van drivers to doctors) to contribute insights and share responsibility for care. Employees are encouraged to consider themselves as part of a team all working toward a common goal—keeping participants happy and healthy. A key to PACE care is proactive primary care—care focused on keeping patients healthy, or at least catching problems early, instead of waiting for problems to develop. This means keeping close tabs on patients. In order to do this, physicians must have access to patients and vice versa. This is usually handled by having physicians officed in the day health care centers. Physicians are salaried PACE employees who work for PACE either full- or half-time. So they have essentially bought into the PACE model.

PACE care does not come cheap. However, this care is supported by payments from both Medicare and Medicaid and PACE is available under Medicare Advantage. In theory, persons not dually covered by Medicare and Medicaid could purchase PACE care privately (in essence paying the Medicaid share), but so far few have taken up that option. Resources providing more information on the development of PACE programs in different parts of the country are available in the appendix.

Assisted Living

For many older people, assisted living can be a wonderful option. Unfortunately, it is frequently overlooked, especially as an immediate option after discharge from a hospital. There are several reasons for this. First, most discharge planners will recommend more traditionally medical environments. Second, assisted living is not covered by Medicare and is tailored toward long-stay care, not rehabilitation. But if you are interested in assisted living, don't let that deter you. It is just as possible to arrange home health care help in an assisted-living facility as in an older person's home.

The assisted-living scene has become more confusing as its popularity has increased. Many providers have rushed in to offer something under this rubric to the point where the term may have lost much of its meaning. It can refer to a coordinated set of services that combines room and board (with greater privacy than a nursing home) with a package of personal-care services, or it can be little more than a residential hotel with a few added amenities.

Assisted-Living Facilities Vary

Not all assisted-living facilities (ALFs) are created equal. But the basic idea behind all ALFs is the same. Assisted living was designed as an alternative option to nursing homes, a way to provide care for frail people in a less institutionalized setting. ALFs address many of the shortcomings of nursing homes. Most ALFs will offer more commodious living situations but substantially less nursing care than nursing homes. They are more likely to have more single rooms and serve better food, usually from a menu of choices.

An ALF typically feels more residential than a nursing home. At the minimum, residents get a single-room apartment, although many units are much more luxurious. The most basic units will have a separate toilet and bath as well as equipment for modest food storage and preparation.

The enthusiasm for assisted living has led people to offer a wide variety of products under that same name. As a result, the buyer must beware. You cannot trust the name to convey what is provided within. Today, the options range from the original models that sought to combine care and independent life to facilities that are little more than scaled-down hotels with a nurse available during the day.

Assisted Living Is Less Regulated Than Nursing Home Care

Assisted living is primarily a privately purchased service, so it is less regulated than nursing home care and more affected by market conditions. Costs and standards vary widely by location. Obviously, the levels of amenities the facility offers will affect the cost. Factors like the size of a person's living space, the lavishness of the surroundings, and the amount of personal service available are all determined by how much they are willing to pay.

Assisted Living and Medicaid

States are increasingly offering assisted living coverage under Medicaid (under what are called waiver programs that allow more discretionary spending), but the levels and types of services vary widely. You should ask about

Medicaid coverage if it is appropriate. Likewise, when speaking to an assisted-living facility, you should ask if they accept Medicaid payment. What will happen if your mother spends out her assets and goes on Medicaid? Too often the ALF will no longer accept her and she will be forced to move out.

Choosing an Assisted-Living Facility

Choosing an ALF involves a lot of research. Unlike with nursing homes, there is no national database to use for preliminary screening. Also, the definition of what is "assisted living" is much more flexible than the definition of "nursing home." There are a wide variety of facilities, providing completely different types and levels of care, and all call themselves "assisted-living facilities."

View the Facility from Your Loved One's Perspective

You need to be very careful as you shop for an ALF. It is important to visit the ALF you are considering. Make sure you conduct the visit cautiously and considerately. Many assisted-living facilities build fancy embellishments to attract families. (A large national chain of ALFs is known for its spiral staircases. These certainly give visitors a sense of grandeur but may be the last way to facilitate frail older people going up and down.) Just because the ALF has a brand-spanking-new fitness center does not mean the facility provides the kind of support you are looking for. Try to look at the place from the perspective of your loved one. The question you should be asking is not, "Would I like to live here?" but rather, "What would living here be like if I were old and frail?"

Beware of Overenthusiastic Salespeople

Because ALFs come in so many shapes and sizes, you must be very diligent if you want to determine what *exactly* you are buying. Much like real estate developers—and many ALFs are in fact run by developers—ALFs often have their own personal sales force. It's important to bear in mind that while these salespeople can be very convincing, they are not the ones who will ultimately provide the care. They can make big promises, because they aren't the ones who have to follow through on them.

If you can, talk with some of the direct care staff. Visit the floors. Nighttime and mealtimes are good times to visit. You may feel a little out-of-place when visiting because you are essentially exploring some-one else's (many other people's, in fact) home. Most residents, how-ever, do not mind your reconnoitering, especially if you engage them in meaningful conversation. This is also a good litmus test for a facility. If staff discourage you from conversing with the residents, that should serve as a warning that this isn't the right place for your older relative. If pos-sible, you should try to talk with family members of current and former residents of the facility you are considering.

When looking for an ALF, be prepared to ask hard questions and demand complete answers. Do not settle for general reassurances. Table 10.4 provides a list of some questions you should ask:

Dealing with Disabilities

You may have noticed that many of the questions on the Assisted Living list address how much care the ALF provides, and how differ-ent disabilities are handled. It is important to make sure you clarify the ALF's policies on these issues. ALF staff's enthusiasm for caring for more disabled people varies widely. Some ALFs view themselves as serving a

Table 10.4: Questions to Ask of Assisted-Living Facilities

What are the criteria for admission? How disabled can a person be physically and/or mentally?
What are the charges for room and board, the facility's basic service package, additional services like hairdressers, medications, and personal-care supplies? What are the fees based on? Are any charges based on a disability assessment? How much personal care is included in the quoted price? Is it calculated by a certain amount of time or by the specific services provided?

Table 10.4 (continued)

What services are included in the basic package? For example, will staff help bathe, dress, and feed residents if they need such assistance? Is that service provided on a temporary or a long-term basis? What is the basis (and charge) for incremental care? How much incremental care is available? What happens if the resident does not need some of the standard services routinely provided by (and charged for by) the facility? What if you want to provide some of those services rather than paying?

What are the facility's activities program like? What kinds of activities are included? Are they designed as diversion or rehabilitation?

How flexible is the ALF's schedule? If a person's former routines are substantially different from the normal practice, how well can the ALF make allowances for that? Can they assist someone in a daily schedule based on their preferences and history (for example, rising time, bathing habits, mealtimes, and bedtime)?

How do they assess and manage psychosocial issues (like anxiety, grief, and aggression)?

How does the facility work with physicians? Does the facility have an on-site medical clinic? Does one physician (or practice) handle the medical needs of the residents, or is each resident expected to find and manage their own care?

What services will the ALF's nursing staff provide? Will they supervise medications? Will they weigh residents? Will they make systematic assessments of specific physiological parameters (such as blood pressure)? Will they oversee changes in medical regimens? Will they assist with bathing and dressing?

How are medications managed? If residents can't manage their own medications even for a short time, how are their medications managed? Who is responsible for ordering, administering, and ensuring that drug interactions and over- or under-medication are avoided?

How much nursing care is available? When and how can a resident request nursing care? How are levels of care established for each resident?

What are the qualifications of the staff? How many have had formal gerontology or geriatrics training? What are the qualifications of the administrator and director of nursing? Is nursing directed by a registered nurse or a licensed practical nurse?

Who decides when a resident's necessary level of care has changed and how to respond to it? Are family members involved in these discussions and decisions? At a minimum, will they be notified of changes in care routines? For example, when weight changes or behavioral changes are noted, who is notified? Does the facility have a system in place to make systematic observations and respond to changes?

If a potential resident needs more care than is typically provided, how can that care be arranged? How is the extra care charged? Can the ALF staff provide it or do you need to hire your own personal aide? Can you purchase the part-time services of an aide who already is on staff, or do you have to hire your own staff separately? Do you have to hire through a prescribed agency, or may you find, hire, and fire your own supplemental staff?

Table 10.4 (continued)

What training (or supervision) does the staff have in working with people with cognitive impairment?
What are the ALF's discharge criteria and practices? How disabled can a person be and still remain a resident? Are some types of behavior automatic grounds for discharge? How do they manage people with dementia?
Is there a separate area for residents with severe cognitive impairment, such as residents with late stage Alzheimer's disease (these are often are called special care units)? What are the criteria for entry into these areas? On the flip side, what are the criteria and supports that make it possible for residents to stay out of these areas?
Does the facility have a nursing home as part of its campus? Do the staff refer residents to a certain nursing home when the resident's needs outstrip the ALF's capacity? What is the ALF's financial relationship to this home?
What happens if a resident runs out of money? How much notice does the family receive? What happens when a family is unable to pay the resident's fees? What is their policy toward accepting Medicaid?
How are emergencies managed? What are the criteria for calling the EMS?

basically functional clientele, people who need only a little assistance at most. This clientele is looking for a living situation that takes care of little tasks like cooking and cleaning. This kind of ALF is more like a retirement hotel. Facilities that prefer to handle a relatively healthy and independent clientele will discharge residents when they become a burden. But other ALFs will really extend the care they provide for an increasingly frail resident. Sometimes these facilities go beyond their capacity to provide adequate care.

Because there is such a spectrum of attitudes, it is important to understand an ALF's policies on disabilities, as well as relevant state policies around admission and discharge criteria. These issues can vary widely from one state to another as well. Remember to ask crucial questions like how do they handle the need for more supportive care? Do they require you to hire your own private duty staff? When do they recalculate the rates? What is the turnover rate for administrators and directors of nursing?

Understand the ALF's Ground Rules

The ground rules for what is covered and what is done vary widely across ALFs and by geographic region. Some, but by no means all, of the variation can be traced to regulation differences. It is important to ascertain the ground rules. When you are interviewing the ALF staff, you need to understand precisely what the criteria are for retention or discharge. Remember key questions like what kinds of changes in status would prompt the facility to push to discharge or relocate the resident. How well does the staff monitor residents' behavior or changing needs? Do they look for the origins of these changes and for possible solutions? How is the family notified when a person's care level has changed? Some enlightened ALFs have the surge capacity to assign more staff when needed. They essentially include the cost of adding more staff "as needed" as part of their overall rate setting. But other ALFs require that families hire additional nurse's aides on their own. You don't want to be surprised by this down the road. Make sure you have all the information before you commit.

Chapter Ten—Points to Ponder

Respect the older people's wishes and desires. Identify what is truly key to their happiness. Reconsider your own risk aversion.

Be realistic and honest about what each option has to offer and how it fits with your overall goals.

Nursing homes can be very restrictive; selecting a high-quality nursing home is an exhaustive process (see Chapter Eleven).

CCRCs fit some older people's needs, but you need to evaluate them carefully.

Assisted living sounds good, but it means so many different things to different people. Buyers must beware.

Eleven

Nursing Homes

THE IMPORTANCE OF OPTIMISM

I vividly recall a lovely ninety-three-year-old woman who came to live at the nursing home where I worked. She had never married, but she had raised a nephew for her brother when his wife died. What I remember most is the way that Gertrude leaned forward, listening carefully to hear each word her visitors said to her. Gertrude truly remained interested in life. And believe it or not, she actually left the nursing home several months after she arrived, by the front door, not the back.

—JOANN HOWITZ, CAREGIVER AND PHYSICAL THERAPIST

The very term "nursing home" is a misnomer. Nursing homes provide little nursing (the vast majority of care is rendered by minimally trained aides), and living conditions are anything but homelike. Most nursing homes are run as institutions. Everyone goes to bed at the same time (usually very early) and gets up at the same time (usually very early) in order to eat (or be fed) at the same time. Meal choices are limited and the food is often tasteless. I have never

understood why regulators are so overly concerned that the food be prepared under a dietician's supervision but not that it taste good. Activities
are uninspired and impersonal. (How much bingo can you stand?) But
the reality is that nursing home stays are common stops for those who
live into their eighties. This means we are all charged with the task of
educating ourselves about the current norms in nursing home care, and
pledging ourselves to seeking continuous improvements in institutional
life for our older loved ones.

History of Nursing Homes

Nursing homes actually began as boardinghouses. Families took in
older people to look after them in addition to their own relatives. But

NURSING HOME LOVE STORIES

In the skilled nursing home where I worked as a physical therapist, I was witness
to some of the greatest love stories I have ever seen. I saw a husband who visited
his wife three times a day for years, even though she could only blink her eyes
to communicate. He watched very carefully to see that she got the proper care.

I saw a son who visited his nearly blind mother for dinner every evening. The
son brought her an appetizer and set up some classical music for her to enjoy
while she ate.

I saw daughters who doted on their mothers and fathers, and saw that their
parent was taken care of even though they as caregivers never received any
thanks.

I saw dietary staff who fried chicken three times a day because that was
the only food that one resident would eat. That same staff went out of their way
every day to try to please residents who had no appetite.

I saw many gentle, kind caregivers who worked at bringing joy and laughter
into the lives of the residents.

—JOANN HOWITZ, CAREGIVER AND PHYSICAL THERAPIST

they eventually became an industry. The big catalyst was the passage of Medicaid. There was now a formal way to pay for such care. With that public payment came the demand for regulations. When today's "modern" nursing homes were first developed, they were designed essentially as mini-hospitals (literally designed after blueprints of small rural hospitals).

Those hospital roots still show in nursing home care today, especially in the rooming structure. Most nursing homes have double-occupancy rooms. Nursing home operators will sell you a load of expensively developed rhetoric praising the idea of sharing a room, but the truth is that most people want single rooms. Who wants to share a room with a stranger? Would you? Probably not. Single rooms provide more privacy and a greater control of your environment, two things most people enjoy. I used to love to uncover the hypocrisy behind the nursing home operators' rhetoric. When I gave speeches to nursing home operators, I would pretend to read a communiqué from the hotel. "I regret to tell you this," I would say, "but the hotel is overbooked, and they're requiring that each of us share a room with the person to our right." The initial horror that followed the announcement clearly illustrated just how highly Americans value privacy and hate the idea of living with strangers. Slowly the nursing home industry is acknowledging this reality.

Single Rooms and the Nursing Home Culture Change

The move toward single rooms is one example of the "culture change" currently gripping nursing homes across the country. Especially with the pressure of competition from assisted living, there is movement afoot to make nursing homes more livable. This reform is occurring in many different ways. Some places are trying to give residents more power by letting them determine their own schedules and menus, for instance. Others have invested in major redesigns of their facilities, building more private rooms. Still others are forming "communities" or "neighborhoods" of ten to fifteen people within the home. These residents are encouraged to work collectively to choose their meals, set their schedules, and generally play an active role in their own and each others' lives.

The development of neighborhood and household models where much of the daily activity takes place in space near the residents' rooms is another kind of reform. The idea is to avoid the cacophony in large dining rooms and the long walks to get to centralized spaces; a goal is also to assign specific staff permanently to a household and a group of residents to ensure that residents experience continuity. The motto of many such organizational structures could be "Small Is Beautiful."

Green Houses

Green Houses is a trademarked term for a radically transformed nursing home that adheres to many principles of neighborhoods but drastically alters the reporting and power relationships. These are comprised of collections of small buildings. Each one houses ten to twelve residents in what is often referred to as a household. The goal is to encourage interactions and friendships. The space is designed to minimize walking distances and encourage congregating in a central living space. The position of nurse aide is transformed into a more universal resident assistant (RA). These workers are responsible for a wide range of tasks including personal care, cooking, and even cleaning. Residents are encouraged to participate in activities like cooking (to the extent that regulations permit).The idea behind Green Houses is to create a more independent community where residents form closer attachments to staff and each other. The concept is still being refined, but it is a real-time illustration of the ways that nursing homes are trying to reinvent themselves.

To use the term Green House, a provider must be part of a consortium that gives permission to use the trademark. Similar "small house" programs are now emerging based on many of the same principles of Green House.

Physician's Role in Nursing Home Care

Time and again, the problems with long-term care come back to bad communication. For example, when doctors and nursing homes communicate poorly with patients and their families, as well as with each other, orders get misunderstood and early signs of problems can be ignored. The challenge is even worse between nursing homes and emergency rooms. Nursing home residents get sent to the hospital with bare-bones information and returned to the home without clear instructions for a continued regimen.

Doctors may even avoid seeing nursing home residents because the staff members communicate so poorly. Middle-of-the-night phone calls with incoherent descriptions of a patient's situation are not likely to endear a particular nursing home to the answering doctor. And the doctor will inevitably take the easiest route, namely sending the patient to the emergency room. (See Chapter Eight.) Physicians are used to working with professional nurses who speak their language and anticipate their needs. Dealing with lesser-trained aides can frustrate them.

A vicious cycle gets rolling. If doctors don't like being in nursing homes, they spend as little time there as possible, rushing through rounds and communicating only briefly with residents or staff. The distance between nursing home staff and the doctor grows harder to bridge. Breaking the cycle requires two things: first, finding clinicians who enjoy working in the nursing home environment, and second, helping nursing home staff to communicate more effectively with the physicians.

As a caregiver in the role of helping to choose a nursing home for a loved one, or continuing to care for a loved one after she enters a nursing home, your best tools are going to be the ability to recognize and not deny the challenges of nursing home care, and being the best advocate you can be for the person you love.

SOMETIMES THE CARING OF A SINGLE STAFF MEMBER CAN MAKE A HUGE DIFFERENCE

When my wife was in the nursing home one nurse's aide gave her special attention. We discussed Ada's condition and ourselves. Often Angie was in Ada's room attending to her when I arrived, and we could talk more freely about our children, our lives, and our problems. She would also, in some of her rare free moments, sit down and chat to me instead of other aides.

Eventually it became apparent that Ada and Angie had a real relationship with each other, so that even when I and others could not get her to smile, if Angie came along, knelt down, and said, "Hi, sweetie," Ada would light up like a candle! It never seemed to fail, and I realized that Angie was a very special person with a unique, loving relationship to my dear wife. As our children visited, they too got to know Angie as a friend. Over the years we all became very close, and we depended upon Angie to help keep us in touch with Ada's gradually deteriorating condition.

Angie attended Ada's memorial service and spoke movingly of her relationship to Ada, and to me and the children. She also spoke eloquently at the nursing home service for residents who had died that month.

—EVILLE GORHAM, CAREGIVING HUSBAND

Choosing the Best Nursing Home

Once you decide that a nursing home is the best care option for your loved one, you are faced with the important task of finding the right nursing home. First and foremost, you must define the preferences and priorities you can agree upon with your loved one and your other family members. What aspects of a nursing home are most important to all of you? Some of these may be absolute and nonnegotiable. For example, a place with a poor quality record is unacceptables however convenient and attractive it is. Take a second to look back at Table 10.1 on page 259. It is time to look into the characteristics of each of your long-term care options.

Cost and Convenience

For most, cost and convenience are the top two most important factors. If your loved one is eligible for Medicaid, it's generally reasonable to look for a home that accepts Medicaid. Nursing homes located nearby are obviously more convenient than those farther away. So location is definitely important. Caregiving does not stop with institutionalization. Older people want to be visited. They will benefit greatly from having someone who can be there regularly to see what is going on and advocate for them. More frequent visits will likely prompt better care and more attention from staff.

Ideally, a nursing home located near the rest of the family, or that part of the family most likely to visit, will lead to more frequent visits. Although most people want to be located where their families are most likely to visit them, and visit them often, experts warn about being swayed too much by a convenient location. A nearby nursing home that provides substandard care is not good enough. And no matter how sincerely family members promise to visit faithfully, the truth is that an unattractive facility or one where the care is poor will decrease the amount of time family members are willing to spend there.

Quality

An important third factor is quality, which includes both quality of care and quality of life. We all like to think we take quality into account when choosing a method of long-term care. However, most people do not really probe the issue directly. Too many people assume that licensing and regulations assure quality. Unfortunately, that is not really true. Far too many substandard facilities continue to operate within the admittedly heavily regulated nursing home industry. And even if you do seriously look into the quality of a nursing home, facilities and care providers change over time and must be reassessed.

If you have found a nursing home in a convenient location, start looking into the quality of care and the kinds of amenities available at that home. Basic information about nursing homes is available on the Web through a federally operated program called Nursing Home Compare (the link for this website is included in the appendix). This program includes virtually all the Medicare-certified nursing homes in the country. You can use the program to find essential information on several quality parameters. In addition, a number of states now publish online their own nursing home report cards, which often provide more detailed information. You can usually access this information by looking up the state's department of health on the Web. They are charged with inspecting nursing homes. Every nursing home is required to post the results of their last state inspection survey. You should at least glance at that to see if there are egregious problems, but passing an inspection does not guarantee a livable environment.

Availability

Another factor of concern is which homes have immediate availability. Depending on the urgency of your situation, you may need to take the care that is available now. For instance, if the hospital is pressing to discharge the patient, you may not have the time for the in-depth research that should be involved in your nursing home decision. Sometimes it's

WHAT IF THE ONLY OPEN HOME IS NOT A GOOD ONE?

If you have no choice but to place your loved one in a substandard nursing home, don't panic. Take the available room, and plan on changing caregivers or locations later if need be. The danger in settling for a subpar home with the intention of moving later is inertia. Once you have made a move for your loved one, it may be hard to summon the effort to move again, but it is misguided to leave an older person in a bad place, even when people tell you about transfer trauma. The problems caused by moves have generally been exaggerated, especially if some efforts are taken to prepare the older person for the move.

possible to place your loved one in a skilled care facility under Medicare while more permanent arrangements are developed. This can give you more time to find the best nursing home. But beware of inertia. Once you have made a move, it takes a lot of effort to mobilize for the next one. That extra effort is usually worth it.

Cost and Coverage of Nursing Home Care

After convenience, cost will probably have the greatest effect on your choice of nursing homes. This is unavoidable. If you are using some form of third-party coverage to pay for care, then your choices will be restricted to the service providers the plan covers. And if you are paying for the care privately, costs may be an even bigger consideration. Older people often are reluctant to spend money for care. They prefer to save their money so that they can leave a financial legacy for their loved ones. Some family members encourage that belief, and see care expenditures as a drain on their inheritance. Major family fights over money are all too common.

Financial Issues to Discuss

When addressing financial issues, as with all aspects of long-term care, up-front honesty (within the family) is absolutely required. First, whose money is involved? Are family members prepared to spend "their" inheritance? Are you prepared to subsidize private care or would you prefer to take advantage of public programs as soon as possible? Even financially well-off older adults may resist spending money on their own care. Some may prefer to make use of public resources (see the section on divestiture in Chapter Two); but many still consider Medicaid as a form of welfare with a heavy stigma attached.

Generally, older people will forgo care because they feel that the needs of younger family members should come first (expenses like college tuition, for example), or they feel that spending their savings threatens the possibility of leaving a legacy. However, if an older person is not eligible for public aid, and chooses to forgo care rather than spend money, you should intervene. Be warned: It may take considerable persuasion to convince your parent to tap into their reserve funds, so be polite but persistent. Another option, which requires some planning and a lot of paperwork, is to advance the funds yourself, as a lien on the older person's estate. Such an arrangement requires cooperation from all potential legatees.

Assessing Quality

As noted, one good way to screen nursing homes is to use Nursing Home Compare, the computerized system developed by the Centers for Medicare and Medicaid Services. This Web-based tool allows you to look up homes by location and to see information about different quality-of-care markers. For instance, you can see how they did on recent surveys and look at the credentials of their staff. Nursing Home Compare shouldn't be used as a be-all and end-all indicator of quality, however. It should be used as a screener, a time-saver. If a home scored poorly, you can probably cross it off your list. But this isn't a vice-versa situation. Just because a home scored well doesn't necessarily mean that the facility is a desirable place to live.

State Report Cards

Depending on where you or your loved one live, you might be able to narrow down your list even further. A number of states publish online "report cards" on nursing homes that provide more information than Nursing Home Compare. Several states also conduct satisfaction surveys of nursing home residents (and sometimes family members) and publish the results.

Hiring an Expert

If your time is at a premium, you may want to hire an expert to help you. A case manager (or care manager) should know each facility within his or her service territory. They should certainly know more than what is posted on Nursing Home Compare. A good case manager can narrow your search by telling you which homes are better than others. They can get on the phone and find out which ones have beds available. A case manager can really streamline the process for you, but at the end of the day, they cannot do the whole job. (See Chapter Nine.)

Make Sure You Visit the Home in Person

By far the most important part of assessing a nursing home is to go there. Visiting is the best way to find out about a nursing home. There is no substitute for seeing the place yourself. Admittedly, that will take time and effort and may be emotionally challenging, but it is worth it.

Visit Unannounced at Multiple Times of Day

You should try to visit at several different times of the day, and unannounced if possible. Two crucial times to visit are at night and during mealtimes. These are among the most stressful times of day for nursing home staff, so you will be able learn a lot about how the staff behaves in trying situations. One good clue is whether both these functions (eating and going to bed) seem to occur for everyone at the same time or whether the home tries to individualize care schedules. When visiting at night, keep an eye on how the staff responds to call bells. Do they react quickly or do they continue watching television and wait for a commercial break? Do they treat residents with respect or chide them for being incontinent? When visiting at mealtimes, check to see if the staff tries to get food into residents as quickly as possible. Do they interact with the residents? Do they take time to talk with them? Are residents lined up in the corridor in wheelchairs? What does the food look like? Some homes are very concerned about choking and make almost everyone eat soft foods. Try some. How does it taste? It will not taste as good as home cooking, but even a little extra care with cooking can make a big difference for a resident who will be eating three meals a day there.

A comprehensive list of issues to look into when choosing a nursing home has been developed by the Legal Services program of Bet Tzedek in Los Angeles. An adapted version of this list is shown as Table 11.1.

PATIENT PREFERENCES MATTER

I had worked in a skilled nursing facility and saw some of the excellent care that residents received. My mother, unfortunately, was not so lucky. Mom's primary health problem was malnutrition. Dad knew that Mom would eat a cup of soup for lunch. Two things that tasted good to her were root-beer floats and pecan pie. Dad would bring ice cream and root beer to the nursing home but the dietary department would not make them for Mom. My brothers walked in one evening to hear a member of the nursing department hollering at my mother! This was the environment of her last six weeks on this earth.

—JOANN HOWITZ, CAREGIVER AND PHYSICAL THERAPIST

THE SMELL TEST

Another good test is the smell of the place. If a nursing home smells of urine and feces, that is a no-brainer. Some smell of Lysol or other cleaning solutions. Not necessarily unpleasant but not ideal either. What you really want is a place that smells like chicken soup or fresh bread, apple pie, or cookies. (Some facilities have actually learned this lesson and try to have good baking smells when visitors are expected. The same advice realtors give you about selling your house.)

Table 11.1: Nursing Home Checklist

Residents
Are the residents' clothes clean?
Are the residents dressed appropriately for the time of day? For the season of the year?
Are the residents clean shaven? Is their hair combed? Are their nails clipped?

Table 11.1 (continued)

Residents' Rooms
Are the residents' rooms clean?
Is the temperature comfortable? Do the rooms have good ventilation, air conditioning, and individual thermostats?
Is there space for personal items?
Have residents decorated their rooms?
Are private baths and showers provided?
Are bathrooms easily accessible for wheelchairs?
Do bathrooms have grab bars near toilets and bathtubs?
Is there adequate closet space?
Can possessions be kept reasonably secure?
Is a private phone available?
Are call buttons easily accessible from bed? From the bathroom?
Is cable television available?
Staff
Do employees know residents by name?
Do employees show respect to the residents?
Does the staff appear to have enough time to care for residents, or are they frantically running from one task to another?
Is the administrator open to your questions and requests?
Is the facility staff receptive to making accommodations for a resident's individual wants or needs? For example, are residents given any say in the selection of a roommate?
How long have staff members been working at the facility?
For how many hours per day is a registered nurse present at the facility? For how many hours per day is a licensed nurse present?
Are nurse's aides assigned so that they generally work with the same residents each day?

Table 11.1 (continued)

Services and Programs
Are social work services performed by a licensed social worker, or by a minimally trained social services designee?
Does the home have a resident council or family council?
Are special events or holiday parties held for the residents?
Are religious services offered at the facility?
Is transportation available for residents who want to participate in social, religious, or community activities outside the facility? Is this transportation wheelchair-accessible?
Does the facility organize activities and field trips that take into account residents' interests?
Does the facility have private areas for residents to meet with family, visitors, or doctors?
Will the staff provide individualized services for the person seeking nursing facility care? If so, can the administrator or director of nurses explain how the services will be provided, and how the facility will ensure that the services actually are provided?
Can the facility provide physical therapy? Speech therapy? Occupational therapy?
Look at the facility schedule for the month. Is there any variety? Are there any activities that would be of interest to the individual seeking nursing home care?
Prevalence of Restraints
How many of the residents are tied up in a bed or chair?
Do the residents seem overmedicated?
Food
Are the dining room and kitchen clean?
Are there unpleasant odors?
Is the staff patient in assisting residents who can't feed themselves?
Does the food taste good? Smell good? Look good?
How much choice do residents have in the food that they are served?

Table 11.1 (continued)

Will the home provide special diets such as low cholesterol or low salt?
Ask the staff for food the prospective resident prefers. How do the staff members respond?
Look at the menu for the month. Is there variety in the menu, or are a few meals served over and over again?
How is food made available between mealtimes?
Physical Surroundings
Is the facility quiet or noisy?
Does the facility have a safe outside area?
Does the facility have a specific room for therapy services?
Location
Is the facility accessible for the prospective resident's family members and friends?
Is the facility close to the prospective resident's familiar neighborhood?
Opinions of Others
What do current residents say about the facility? What do their family members and friends say?
Does the prospective resident's doctor have an opinion about the facility? Is the prospective resident's doctor willing to visit the resident at the facility?
Payment
Is the facility certified to accept reimbursement from the Medicare program? From the Medicaid program?
Does the facility have a relationship with the resident's health maintenance organization?
What is the daily rate?
What "extra charges" are not included in the daily rate?
Is a deposit required? (Remember, a deposit cannot be required if the resident's care will be covered by Medicare and/or Medicaid.)

Table 11.1 (continued)

Public Records
Are inspection reports easily accessible from the facility?
How many violations (and what kind of violations) have been found by the local licensing and certification agency?
Have monetary fines been assessed against the facility?
Has the facility been threatened with loss of its license, or loss of its federal certification?
Have any lawsuits been filed against the facility?

Source: Bet Tzedek Legal Services and National Senior Law Center, *Nursing Home Companion*, 2003.

Making the Move

Moving a parent into a nursing home can be traumatic. In many cases it means closing up a home that they have lived in for many years. Many older people are reluctant to make this move; some adamantly resist it. Families often resort to subterfuge. They may make it appear that they are just visiting the facility to take a look and then move the older person into a bed, or leave them sitting in a wheelchair. It is easy to see why this tactic may not be a good idea, however desperate things seem.

Know Your Loved One's Wishes for Transferring Belongings

In the best of worlds the decision to move into a nursing home will have come about after careful deliberation and joint discussions. The compromise nature of this solution will be appreciated, and promises made about how to mitigate the adverse effects. Certainly there will be promises of frequent visits. It may be possible to choose some items the older person can bring from home. Some homes may actually allow people to bring in some furniture, but most restrict personal items to smaller things. It will be important to decide how to dispose of the older person's

A DIFFICULT TRANSITION

My bitterest memory is of the ploy used to get my mother into a nursing home. My mother was eighty-six years old. She had a good memory, a frail body, and severe osteoporosis with a spine as out of alignment as any that I have seen. Mom's primary problem was malnutrition.

On the other hand, my eighty-four-year-old dad had early dementia and a good physical body. My dad took such good care of my mother that he brought her things before she knew that she wanted them. I guess that is what happens after you have been married for sixty-four years.

In addition to my parents, my forty-six-year-old mentally challenged sister, Rose, lived with Mom and Dad. Mom could tell Dad and Rose what to do and they could do the physical part. The home and residents were clean at all times, bills were paid, outside assistance was used as needed, and a home-health nurse came to see my mother every week or two. I also visited my parents every other week and talked to them frequently on the telephone.

I was aware of the fact that the home-health nurse did not approve of the situation at my parents' home (and the fact that they lived in a very small farm town only made scrutiny all the more intense). One day I got a telephone call at work from the nurse informing me that my mother must go to the hospital immediately. As I was 150 miles away and could not see the situation, I agreed to the request. The hospital assessed my mother and promptly sent her to the nursing home. There is no doubt in my mind that this was a means of getting Mom out of the house.   —JOANN HOWITZ, CAREGIVER AND PHYSICAL THERAPIST

furniture and belongings. In many cases, they will have very detailed and exacting plans for who should get what. Even if the intended recipients are less than thrilled, it is best to suggest that these benefactions will be met. Both my mother and my mother-in-law made a long list of instructions for the disposition of their property (including some exaggerated estimates of the value of their jewelry). When the time came to dispose of the things, only a few could really be used by those for whom they were intended, but what matters is honoring the person's requests.

Make Moving Day an Event

It is a very bad idea to spring a move on an older person. The idea of suggesting going for a ride and then dropping them off at a nursing home has the same appeal as abandoning a baby at an orphanage doorstep.

On the actual moving day, it is best to make the move an event. Relevant family should attend, perhaps as reassurance that the older person will not be abandoned. Facilities vary in how they handle the intake. Some are content to allow time to settle in and say good-bye. Others like to have new residents quit cold turkey and advise families to stay away for several days to allow for a period of adjustment. There may be some fear that the initial adaptation will be difficult and families will be tempted to renege. I am generally wary of this latter approach.

In the New Home: Families Can Help Their Loved One Adjust

One strategy for families is to play an active role in facilitating the transition. They can help with acclimation by showing the older person where things are.

- Where the dining room is
- Where the pharmacy and/or gift shop are
- Where the cafeteria is
- Where the library is
- Where the activities occur
- Where lounges are
- Where the phone is
- If possible, where his or her room/apartment is
- Where the car will be parked
- Where the mailboxes are
- Where he or she can cash a check

Settling In to the Nursing Home

When thinking about moving into a nursing home, I am often reminded of a version of the French Foreign Legion slogan "Adapt or Die." Certainly

AN INSIDER'S STORY

I was doing the admission physical therapy evaluation on a ninety-one-year-old man. When I asked the gentleman why he came to live at the nursing home, he replied, "I can't see out of one eye and the other eye can't see either." The evaluation progressed and I asked John to go for a walk with me. He picked up his cane and away we went. As we walked in the hall a nurse was standing at her med cart with her back to us. John, the man who could not see, picked up his cane and with perfect aim goosed the nurse. He then turned and gave me a big grin. Yeah right, he could not see!

—JOANN HOWITZ, CAREGIVER AND PHYSICAL THERAPIST

some level of adaptation is necessary, but there are varying ways of adapting. The staff would obviously prefer compliance. The challenge is how to preserve one's sense of self. Nursing homes may be developing a stronger sense of humanity and realizing that there is no mandate that everyone get up at the same time or eat at the same time. Indeed, they are coming to appreciate that there may even be efficiencies in allowing some variation in schedules.

Nursing home residents need to find some way to continue to retain their individual identities. They also need to learn how to fit into a group. Some compromises are necessary. Obviously those with more social skills and those who enjoy the company of others will fare better.

Many older people enter nursing homes because they suffer from dementia. In many instances they may no longer be in touch with their surroundings. Nonetheless they do seem to react to certain stimuli. Environments can influence behavior more than we often appreciate. In some instance, even persons with advanced dementia formed friendships when allowed to interact in conducive environments.

Visiting and Advocacy

A family's work does not stop when an older person is admitted to a nursing home. Shopping to find the right home is important but the job does not end there. There is lots to do when the older person is living there. Families can play proactive roles. For example, some provide a bird feeder right at the window and keep it filled. Families need to know how to visit—they shouldn't go tiptoeing around—they have to remember it is their relative's home first, not the staff's workshop first. They can close the door. They can take their relative for a walk with the wheelchair or walker.

Nursing home residents' well-being depends on visitors. It is vital that nursing home residents not feel abandoned. Residents who are visited may get better care if the staff believes the families are watching what is done. Family members are usually the prime advocates for the residents. They can raise issues with the staff about inadequate care. The more they are there, the more they can observe the quality of the care.

Playing the advocate role can be tricky. While the squeaky wheel gets the grease, you cannot afford to get slathered too often. You are vulnerable because you do not want to trigger some sort of retaliatory action out of sight. Thus, you need to choose your battles carefully. It is a tricky call. Family members who carp about every small infringement and inadequacy may be dismissed when there is a big problem. Conversely, letting everything slide in anticipation of handling the one "really big issue" may not be the best course, either. Balance and judgment are the keys.

One needs to be very skeptical when a nursing home claims that regulations do not allow something. When a NH says "this isn't allowed," ask for details. For example, a woman in Texas complained that the NH where her father was a private pay resident for a year told her and her brother that a new Texas rule prohibited them from taking him out on holidays anymore. That seems like a strange rule. More likely, the NH would have had to reduce the bill for the week her father was on vacation and they didn't want to do it.

Getting Involved in Care Planning

Families should play an active role in planning the care for their older relatives. Typically, the nursing home invites family members to the care planning conference. Family members may feel a little cowed to be sitting among professionals, but the family's input is essential. The decisions made at these care planning sessions are critical, because once a care plan is made, it rules the day. It is very important that family play an active role. The planning process may involve all sorts of minutia. There should also be some discussion of how the family can best work with the nursing home. Whom should they see about what? Protocols will vary among nursing homes but families need to know who organizes transportation, who keeps the accounts for the beauty shop and expenditures, and on and on. They have to understand the nursing hierarchy.

When the Nursing Home Option Fails

Some people are simply not cut out for nursing home life. Usually older people are not sent to nursing homes these days until fairly late in their clinical course, when they may have lost some of their vital energy to resist. They may become passive and compliant. Indeed, this is a typical coping mechanism when placed in a situation where you have little power or control. It is termed "learned helplessness," and often leads to depression.

A tough call is when to decide that this arrangement is not working out. Family relieved of the burdens of daily care may be reluctant to face the evidence that their loved one is declining. But in some cases it may make better sense to set up (or reestablish) a more expensive home care program.

KEEP A FALLBACK OPTION OPEN

In many cases, it may be wise, if possible, not to undo your loved one's prior living situation too quickly upon a move to a nursing home. You do not want to cut off your options if the nursing home arrangement does not work out.

Chapter Eleven—Points to Ponder

Nursing homes should be considered, but only in the context of other options.

Shop carefully. Use Web-based information, but visit, too. Nothing can replace being there. Keep your eyes open when you visit. Don't ignore unpleasant things.

Use the checklist on page 284.

Recognize that the move can be traumatic. Prepare the older person. Do not deceive him.

Visit often. It is too easy to abandon older people in institutions.

Visited people generally get better care.

Advocate deliberately. Choose your battles.

Twelve

End of Life

End-of-life decisions and processes are difficult before, during, and after death. Most people try to deny the reality of impending death as long as possible. (Ironically, family members are more likely to deny death than is the dying person.) Some of it is unfounded optimism; some is raw denial. In the last decades, thinking about the end of life has changed considerably. More and more people are grappling with what is called "futile care." This term applies to treatments offered without real expectations of benefits. Modern life-support technology allows us to keep people alive long after they have effectively died. It allows us to offer expensive, often dangerous, treatments that offer only limited chances of succeeding. But increasing numbers of people are stating their wishes to forgo heroics. They are choosing to concentrate on palliative care—care aimed at ameliorating unpleasant symptoms. Instead of trying to cure their illnesses, they are opting to make the end of their lives as comfortable as possible while not prolonging the process of death.

Talking About Death

End-of-life discussions can be shrouded in religious controversy. But most religions distinguish between allowing people to die a natural death without the use of heroic measures and causing that death to occur sooner than it would have naturally. Most religions—and governments—permit people to forgo extreme measures to prolong their lives. Assisted suicide, however, is still prohibited in most states. Oregon is the only state with a liberal policy on physician-assisted suicide and self-determination. But remarkably, even though those options are available in Oregon, they are rarely used.

Go Easy on Yourself

No matter how well you prepare for a loved one's death or how long the dying process lasts, death is always hard for the survivors. It is important not to beat yourself up. Try to take solace in looking back to appreciate all that you did to make this last stage of life as comfortable as possible for your loved one. But even that will not protect you from the sense of loss. And that is okay. Everyone should be mourned and celebrated. Everyone's life can be a source of lessons about how to live and how not to live one's life.

End-of-Life Decisions

In Chapter Two, we talked about advance directives. To review, advance directives are formal indications of a person's preferences about what types of treatment she would and would not want under various circumstances. Advance directives require a person to make fairly heroic assumptions about what life would be like under different conditions. End-of-life decisions differ from advance directives in that the person is actually experiencing the living condition she could only have speculated about earlier. The older person is facing her fears, so she is in a much better situation to know when she will find living in that state unbearable. Any responsible program for end-of-life care should include in-depth discussions about end-of-life preferences. However, you should never use these discussions to attempt to convince your loved one to opt out of treatment. These discussions should be an opportunity for dying persons to voice their opinions. They should never become opportunities for other people—professionals or family members—to impose their beliefs and preferences on an older patient. Pastoral counselors and social workers can be especially helpful, both by providing support and helping to thoroughly examine end-of-life care options.

Both advance directives and end-of-life decision-making should be seen as opportunities for an older person to expand the role they play in planning their care. This is the time for a dying person to clarify their personal views on treatment benefits and risks; to identify their choices and preferences; and to ensure that those choices and preferences will be executed. In an end-of-life situation, however, it is crucial to remember that advance directives should never be used to override a patient's real-time preferences.

These discussions are often harder for family members to initiate than they are for the older person. Many older people want to talk about the end of their lives and to make plans. At least give them the opportunity.

Hospice Care

Special approaches to end-of-life care can take several forms. One of the more traditional forms is hospice care. Hospice is a specific program designed especially for patients who have a finite prognosis— meaning patients who have six months or less to live. Hospice arose as a response to what many saw as the insensitive way that formal medical care addressed the dying process. Hospice was designed to serve both the patient and the family. Originally, hospice was intended for cancer patients. However, since then it has been expanded to address the needs of people with other diagnoses—advanced heart disease, pulmonary disease, or even dementia. In the United States, the majority of hospice care is provided by volunteers in the patients' private homes. However, regardless of whether hospice care is provided at home or in institutional settings, hospice represents a suspension of the usual rules for medical care. The priority of care is no longer a commitment to preserving life at any cost. Instead, the emphasis shifts to making the patient's last days of life as carefree and pain-free as possible. The usual restrictions on things like visiting hours are typically suspended. Pain medication is used generously, without the (usually misguided) fear of creating addiction.

Hospice and Medicare

Hospice care is available as a specific benefit under Medicare. When a person enrolls in the hospice benefit, they literally shift their coverage for their terminal condition to a new plan and a different kind of care. If they suffer from multiple conditions, they can retain traditional Medicare coverage for other problems. If they are enrolled in Medicare, and they are considering hospice care, make sure to find a Medicare-certified hospice program.

Doctor Certification and Terminal Prognosis

Essentially a Medicare beneficiary signs up for a hospice program. To do so, a doctor must certify that the patient is expected to live less than six months. However, many terminal patients outlive their projected life spans by quite a margin. For people interested in hospice care, the requirement for a terminal prognosis can create problems in two ways. First, many physicians and families are reluctant to make a terminal prognosis. Because most put this off for as long as possible, the average length of a hospice admission is only three weeks. Second, making a terminal prognosis is difficult. When physicians are asked to specifically predict how long a patient has to live, they're prone to substantial error in both directions. One approach to dealing with this problem is to phrase the question differently. Instead of asking how long the doctor thinks the patient will live, ask whether the doctor would be surprised if the patient died in the next six months.

Hospice Supports Death at Home

Hospice care under Medicare is intended as a non-hospital service delivered primarily at home. In some cases, it is provided in nursing homes. Hospice patients can be hospitalized for palliative care and emergencies, but the pricing of the hospice benefit deters heavy use of hospitals. If you opt for hospice care, understand that the goal is that the patient die at home if at all possible.

Medicare/Medicaid Hospice Benefits

Hospice services are reimbursed under Medicare. Under the Medicare/Medicaid Hospice Benefit, patients are eligible for many services not ordinarily covered by Medicare/Medicaid. Services in this benefit may include (as "medically appropriate"):

- Routine registered nurse visits
- Registered emergency on-call nurse
- Doctor services
- Social work services
- Homemaker-home health aide
- Physical, speech, and occupational therapy
- Dietary counseling
- Chaplain and spiritual care
- Bereavement counseling
- Prescription medications
- Medical equipment
- Medical supplies
- Palliative radiation treatment
- Continuous nursing care
- Inpatient short-term care
- Respite care
- Medical transportation

Services Not Covered by Medicare Under the Hospice Benefit May Include:

- Medical care for illness and disease unrelated to terminal illness (regular Medicare or Medical Assistance covers these services)
- Inpatient care in a noncontracted facility
- Twenty-four-hour sitters or caregivers
- Medical transportation (except as arranged by the hospice)
- Over-the-counter medications
- Aggressive or curative treatment

Palliative Care

In recent years, public support for hospice care is giving way to greater support for palliative care. Palliative care takes a broader approach than hospice care. It not only supports those who are dying but also those with chronic conditions who are, in a sense, also dying, albeit more slowly. Palliative care does not require a terminal prognosis. It applies the core concepts of hospice care—life with dignity right up until death with pain and symptom control—but it does not rule out continued active treatment when appropriate.

Comparing Palliative and Hospice Care

In essence, the palliative care approach embraces many of the techniques developed in hospice, but it does not require that the patient or the physician make a formal declaration of terminal status. Indeed, it can be initiated at any point in the course of a life-threatening chronic illness. Palliative care puts the attention on pain management, including emotional pain, as well as managing other symptoms of discomfort (such as itching). Palliative care also seeks to reduce distress among patients and burnout among caregivers. For example, palliative care could allow surgery to relieve a gastrointestinal obstruction, even if the surgery had no hope of improving the overall prognosis. But palliative care doesn't rule out treatment like chemotherapy for cancer or any aggressive approach to treating advanced chronic disease.

Ironies of Hospice and Palliative Care

There is a certain irony to the idea of both hospice and palliative care. In a way, both of these forms of care imply that the process of dying entitles a patient to greater focus on the same distressing symptoms and concerns that might be dismissed as trivial for those with a better chance of survival. That reasoning seems flawed. Why should living people not be made as comfortable as those who are dying? The very fact that we have programs like hospice and palliative care speaks volumes about the shortcomings of contemporary medical care. If you are frustrated by the limitations of our system, make sure to read the final chapter of this book, where I give advice on how you can change that system.

How to End Medical Treatment

At some point it may be necessary to decide that further care is no longer in the patient's best interest. Hopefully by the time families reach this point, conversations have already transpired, at least in principle, about the circumstances of the end of life. It is, in part, the basis for advance directives.

My sister and I talked a great deal about how our mother's quality of life was deteriorating, and that helped us to make the end-of-life decision about when to stop or forgo heroic care. We almost rehearsed what we would do. Nonetheless, when the nursing home called to say that our mother was having trouble breathing and seemed to be slipping away, I agreed to giving her intravenous fluids just in case it might simply be dehydration. However, we drew the line at antibiotics, and she died in two days.

END-OF-LIFE DISAGREEMENTS REQUIRE MEDIATION

If there is family disagreement over discontinuing or forgoing care in an end-of-life situation, some sort of mediation will be needed. Hospital social workers may help, but likely someone trusted by all sides may need to be brought in. Needless to say, such a person must be skilled in family counseling. All sorts of issues are likely to arise.

Family Members Must Be in Consensus

It is critical to achieve family consensus about when further efforts are futile and may cause more suffering than benefit. Collective agreement will (hopefully) prevent later recriminations. Moreover, most institutions will resist any efforts to discontinue care if they feel some family members are opposed, because they fear malpractice suits.

It Isn't Over When It's Over

Even after your loved one dies, some vestiges of caregiving remain. There are bills to be paid and accounts to be closed. Some of these responsibilities persist for quite a while. One individual who gives advice on aging and other topics in a regular radio program found herself struggling years after her mother's death to settle bills with a home care company. She'd thought that her mother was on Medicaid, and that they were covering the costs. Unfortunately, the patient's enrollment process had become derailed somehow, and now the daughter was left to straighten out the mess long after her mother's passing. First of all, she needed to establish her deceased mother's Medicaid status. Then she needed to clarify her financial responsibility for the costs of her mother's care. Needless to say, this was not the easiest way for her to cope with the grieving process. Her first step was to find a lawyer with a record in elder law, but such help does not come cheap. Ultimately, this woman ended up spending a significant amount of money on resolving a care situation that no longer directly aided anyone.

Healthy Grieving

One important task is grieving. While grieving is a natural state, denial is not. Therefore, it is best to expect and accept the negative and difficult emotions that accompany the loss of a loved one. Death is associated with pain and loss. That is why we have created rituals like funerals and memorial services to help deal with this emotion. Religion plays a strong role in easing this burden for many people, but certainly not all.

Dangers of Grief

Grieving can be a dangerous time. Spousal deaths (especially among men) are high in the six months after bereavements. Families need to be mindful of what happens to the surviving spouse and prevent an inordinate period of grieving. Life must go on.

Grief manifests in many different ways. Some of the responses to grief include:

- Difficulty accepting your loss
- Deep sorrow
- Irritability and moodiness
- Sleeplessness
- Depression and/or anxiety
- Guilt
- Anger
- Fear
- Lack of motivation
- Social withdrawal
- Obsessive thoughts of your loved one
- Eating too much or too little
- Fatigue

- Physical pain or illness
- Intense dreams or nightmares

Grieving should be a transitional state. The active symptoms should not last more than six months. If these symptoms persist after that period, you should be concerned about more serious emotional problems and you should seek professional help.

Chapter Twelve—Points to Ponder

Advance directives are different from end-of-life decisions.

Living wills are more restrictive than durable powers of attorney.

Do not be afraid to talk about the end of life, with the older person and with the rest of your family.

Avoid futile care.

Consider hospice care early.

Recognize the dangers of excessive grieving.

Thirteen

Political Advocacy

Getting the System We Want and Need

Most of this book is designed to help individual families cope with the challenges and surprises of caring for an aging loved one. However, no matter how skilled a practitioner of case management science you are, you can accomplish only so much alone. I learned that lesson all too well when I helped organize care for my own mother.

Much of the public discussion about long-term care has emphasized how to pay for it, but that misspecifies the problem. My mother never relied on Medicaid. It was not a matter of paying for her care; the challenge was finding the kind of care we wanted to pay for. Even with all that I knew and all my connections, I found it very difficult to get the care I thought she deserved. In the end, I concluded that the problem was not in how I was working with the system, it was in the system itself. The system needs to become easier to use and more effective in meeting the needs of older people. We are the ones who are losing out on this issue. If we want to the system to get better, we need to collectively demand changes.

Historically, advocacy for frail older people has been weak. Groups that might be expected to provide leadership, like AARP, focus more on issues that concern healthier older people—things like Social Security and Medicare, the marketing of insurance products, and prescription drugs. The natural advocates of older people are their families, especially those who have been caught up in the struggle to get good long-term care for their parents and spouses. In stark contrast to advocacy on behalf of younger persons with disabilities, many of whom have lifelong supporters, advocacy on behalf of frail older people is ephemeral at best. Once an older person dies, the family usually tries to put the whole unpleasant experience behind them. Apart from disease-based organizations (like the Alzheimer's Association), long-term care has never attracted a sustained group of supporters willing to work to improve the situation. The advocacy that does exist is usually driven by care providers, rather than care consumers.

Misconceptions About Long-Term Care

I believe there are several reasons for this general lack of advocacy, but here are the three big misconceptions that deter a more aggressive effort to improve long-term care:

Good long-term care does not make a difference in the end.

This is a widespread misconception. Because long-term care is associated with a general pattern of decline, there is a certain feeling of hopelessness and helplessness. Many caregivers erroneously believe nothing can be done to prevent the inevitable. The basic measure of success for long-term care is that it slows the unavoidable decline. This makes it hard to easily show people the difference good care can make.

Ironically, long-term care is an area where small differences can produce enormous gains. Good care can make the quality of a person's life better and give them a greater ability to function. Good care can also help caregivers. Early attention to medical problems lets you avoid expensive and destructive catastrophes that require large amounts of care and cost.

The ultimate goal of long-term care should be keeping older people out of hospitals. With a good care system, this end could be so much more achievable.

If I have enough money, good care will not be a problem.

Long-term care is closely tied to welfare. Much of the cost of long-term care is paid by Medicaid, so it has become synonymous with welfare and been tarred with the same brush. Welfare programs do not draw the same kind of concern that middle-class programs do. What many people do not realize is that people covered by Medicaid may be better off than those trying to navigate the system on their own. You might think using your own money will give you more choices about how to purchase care, but the trade-off is that you'll have less guidance. In some cases, you might actually have less access to care resources.

My mother had enough money to buy care, but we could not find the care we wanted to buy. New proposals are calling for consumer-directed care under Medicaid. In effect, Medicaid beneficiaries who need long-term care would have an option of taking cash in lieu of covered services and buying their own care. They will them find themselves in much the same situation my sister and I were in with our mother. Some people predict that there will be a dramatic market response to all this new cash, but I am less inclined to believe that the market will spontaneously create the needed services. Indeed, they will sell services but not necessarily the right ones.

It is time to make good long-term care a common cause. We need to work collectively to improve the long-term care system. Everyone has a stake in this issue—old people, adult children, young family members who do not receive all the time and resources they crave, taxpayers, and professionals. Long-term care affects virtually every family in America at some time. The buying power of a collective market should be able to convince care providers to provide the kinds of care people really want.

Old people are not as important as young people.

Ageism is still alive and well in America. Economists have adopted a measure of program efficiency based on something called quality-adjusted life-years (QALYs). In essence, this measure implies that people with less life expectancy and those who suffer disability have less valuable lives and should be discounted when calculating the value of a given treatment. Under this assumption, frail older people are double losers. Are we really prepared to say that the value of a year of a person with disability's life is worth half that of an able-bodied person?

Even controlling for disability, we all operate under a double standard. Care options that we see as essential for younger people with disabilities aren't actively considered for frail older people. Most agree that younger people with disabilities should have personal-care attendants to enable them to participate fully in all phases of life. And at the same time, we're still content to warehouse older people in institutions, forcing them to share rooms with strangers and live by other people's rules. Is it really surprising that all too often these older people lose their will to live? We deprive older people of their independence in the false name of safety and protection. We deny older people the right to take risks because they're doddery and vulnerable. But why should they not have the opportunity to live on their own if that is what they wish? Why should they not be allowed to forgo care if they do not want to endure the discomfort and sacrifices of the treatment?

I am always amazed that a young person can climb a mountain without a rope and be covered by health insurance if she falls, but an older person is not allowed to walk across a room for fear of falling.

The rampant ageism in our society is aided and abetted by older people as well. Many older people have come to believe that they are not entitled certain things simply because they are old. They believe it is right to discriminate on the basis of age. Older people are reluctant to crusade for their rights. Instead, they accept second-class status and the poor services that come with it.

What to do?

Those three reasons are part of hundreds of others. People have complex and unpredictable reactions to developing disabilities. One serious complicating factor in the battle for equal rights for seniors is that most older people do not want to be a burden on their children. They will suffer all kinds of deprivation to avoid living with their children or imposing on them for assistance.

Children often have a hard time accepting that fact, and American society is ambivalent about the family's role in care. This makes some older people unwilling to accept help. They may try to hide their situations out of pride. Or maybe because they are worried that their decision-making power will be taken from them or that they will be institutionalized. Each older person reacts to disability in their own way. Some accept and adapt; others struggle against it and reject help.

Many people see the so-called baby boomer generation as both a danger and an opportunity. This generation is a demographic tsunami that threatens to engulf the care system when it hits old age. Some forecasters predict that this generation will demand better care and more consumer-oriented changes in the system with their sheer strength of numbers. But I say that the baby boomers can have the most impact now, as the caregivers of their parents. I am not convinced that frail baby boomers with dementia will be any more forceful than their parents have been in advocating on their own behalfs. If they are the consumer force they are portrayed as, they will demand better care for their parents. Their actions today will shape the care they themselves receive tomorrow.

In order to be effective, the boomers need to act at two levels. First, they need to use the force of the marketplace to shape provider responses to care demands. They can do this by insisting on getting both quality of care and quality of life, and not accepting a false trade-off. Second, they must become a political force. They need to push a long-term care agenda that supports access to good care for all—regardless of how it is paid for. The nation is talking about health care right now. Long-term care advocates cannot let this opportunity slide.

If we want to fix the long-term care system, we need to start with the way it is regulated. Current regulations stop the system from providing better care. Undoubtedly, the system needs standards, but overregulation limits innovation just when it is sorely required. Regulations play a role in preventing serious care abuses, but they can also constrain good care. Punishing bad care doesn't motivate good care. Rewards must be mixed with punishment. We need new methods that provide incentives for better care at every level. We should emphasize rewarding organizations that achieve exceptional results, measured in terms of both quality of care and quality of life.

Appendix

ADDITIONAL RESOURCES BY CHAPTER

Chapter Two: The Money and the Law
More information on Medicare Part D:
www.medicare.gov/medicarereform/drugbenefit.asp

More information on Medicare Advantage:
www.medicareadvocacy.org
www.aging.state.ks.us/SHICK/Managed_Care/Disenrollment.htm

More information on private long-term care insurance:
www.naic.org (click on "Long-Term Care Insurance: What You Should Know")

More information on the Vial of Life Project:
www.vialoflife.com

Five Wishes
www.agingwithdignity.org/five-wishes.php

Chapter Three: Finding a Good Doctor
Contact information for the American Geriatrics Society:
Tel. 212-308-1414
www.americangeriatrics.org/contact.shtml

Chapter Four: Caring for Yourself

Support groups:

www.caregiving.com

Alzheimer's Association: www.alz.org/index.asp

Index of disease-specific organizations (e.g., Arthritis Foundation, American Heart Association)

Chapter Five: Daily Life

More information on safer homes:

www.healthyagingprograms.org

Chapter Six: Common Ailments and Treatments

Online symptom checker:

www.webmd.com

Chapter Seven: The Aging Brain

More information on Alzheimer's disease:

www.memorylossdvd.com

www.alzheimersrxtreatment.com/caregiving.html

Chapter Eight: Handling Hospitals

More information on the rights of hospital patients:

www.hcqualitycommission.gov, website of the Advisory Commission on Consumer Protection and Quality in the Health Care Industry

www.aha.org/aha/ptcommunication/partnership/index.html, website of the American Hospital Association (AHA)—The Patient Care Partnership: Understanding Expectations, Rights and Responsibilities

Chapter Nine: Send Help!

More information on Home Instead and their selling tactics:

www.home-instead.com

www.consumeraffairs.com/age/aging.htm

Contact information for case manager certifying organizations:

www.cmsa.org

www.cfcm.com

www.socialworkers.org/credentials/specialty/c-swcm.asp

How to find a case manager:

Call your local local AAA at (800-510-2020)

Or go to one of these websites:
www.RNCaseManager.com
www.SWCaseManager.com
www.cmrg.com
www.caremanager.org
www.findacaremanager.org
www.nia.nih.gov/HealthInformation/Publications/LongDistanceCaregiving/
    chapter06.htm
www.longtermcarelink.net/a2bfindmanager.htm
www.eldercare.gov/Eldercare.NET/Public/Home.aspx
www.n4a.org

Chapter Ten: Moving Time
More information on PACE:
www.cms.hhs.gov/QualityInitiativesGenInfo/10_PACE.asp
www.npaonline.org/website/article.asp

Chapter Eleven: Nursing Homes
Nursing Home Compare:
www.medicare.gov/NHCompare

Chapter Twelve: End of Life
How to find legal assistance:
www.naela.org, National Academy of Law Attorneys (NAELA)
www.aadmm.com, American Association of Daily Money Managers
www.aarp.org, American Association of Retired Persons (AARP)

General end-of-life resources:
www.caringinfo.org
www.caregiver.org
www.caregiving.com
www.nfcacares.org
www.familycaregiving101.org
www.abcd-caring.org
www.hospicefoundation.org
www.healthfinder.gov
www.alz.org
www.sharethecare.org
www.caregiver.org/caregiver

General Information:
The newsletter *Life Ledger Caregiving Tips* is available by paid subscription
mailbox@elderissues.com

A LIST OF RESOURCES

AARP Internet Resources, www.aarp.org/internetresources, a wonderful, frequently updated warehouse resource for websites about aging.

AARP's list of senior websites, www.aarp.org/cyber/general.htm, a comprehensive listing including all members of Congress, lots of state contacts, etc.

AccentCare, www.accentcare.com, provides a wide range of caregiving services that enable seniors to live independently at home.

Aging Research and Education Center, University of Texas Health Sciences Center at San Antonio, www.uthscsa.edu/AREC, one of the preeminent research programs in aging and geriatrics in the nation.

Aging Solutions, www.aging-parents-and-elder-care.com, gives advice, comprehensive checklists, and links to key resources—designed to make it easier for family caregivers to quickly find the information they need and avoid missing things that are important for the care of their loved one.

American Association of Homes and Services for the Aging, www.aahsa.org, provides information about different types of homes and services for the aging and information on careers in aging services. Listings of homes for the aging in every state appear on the association's website.

American Federation on Aging, www.infoaging.org: "Knowledge we all need to live healthier, longer lives."

American Society on Aging, www.asaging.org, the largest network of professionals in the field of aging.

Area Agencies on Aging, www.aoa.gov/AoARoot/AoA_Programs/OAA/How_To_Find/Agencies/find_agencies.aspx, provided by the Administration on Aging.

Benefits CheckUp, www.benefitscheckup.org, a helpful site by the nonprofit National Council on the Aging; guide to state and federal programs helping seniors and caregivers.

Caregiver Magazine, www.caregiver.com, Caregiver Media Group (Today's Caregiver Magazine, Caregiver.com, etc.) and all of its products are developed for caregivers, about caregivers, and by caregivers.

Center for Healthy Aging, www.centerforhealthyaging.org, a nonprofit organization whose mission is to meet the needs of aging adults and their families.

Consumer Consortium on Assisted Living, www.ccal.org, the only national consumer-focused advocacy organization dedicated solely to the needs and rights of assisted-living residents.

Elder Law Answers, www.elderlawanswers.com, a site with good legal information and more for seniors and the elderly.

Eldercare Locator, www.eldercare.gov, U.S. service to find programs and supportive services to help people care for an older member of their family in their homes and communities.

Health and Age, www.healthandage.com, Novartis Foundation on Gerontology site with lots of information on senior health.

Hospice Patients Alliance, www.hospicepatients.org, provides information about hospice services and directly assists patients, families, and caregivers in resolving difficulties they may have with current hospice services, and promotes better-quality hospice care.

Long Term Care Link, www.longtermcarelink.net, a comprehensive noncommercial source of long-term care information.

Medicare News Watch, www.medicarenewswatch.com, Medicare news for beneficiaries, caregivers, and health care professionals.

National Adult Day Services Association, www.nadsa.org, a directory of adult day-care centers and links to other related sites.

National Council on the Aging (NCOA), www.ncoa.org, the nation's first national nonprofit group of people and organizations dedicated to promoting the dignity, independence, well-being, and contributions of older people.

National Council of Senior Citizens, www.ncscinc.org, works to improve the lives of the elderly and people of all ages.

Program of All-Inclusive Care for the Elderly (PACE), www.npaonline.org, helps provide and coordinate all needed preventive, primary, acute, and long-term care services so older individuals can continue living in the community.

Senior Journal, www.seniorjournal.com/index.html, "Today's News and Information for Senior Citizens and Baby Boomers."

State Agencies on Aging, www.eldercare.gov/eldercare.net/public/network/ sua.aspx, provided by the Administration on Aging.

State Legal Assistance for the Elderly, www.ilrg.com/practice/assistelderly.html.

Federal Government

All-in-one government site, www.firstgov.gov, from which you can reach all government sites and information.

Administration on Aging, www.aoa.gov, information from the federal agency that deals with issues affecting older Americans.

Aging Initiative, www.epa.gov/aging, a site by the Environmental Protection Agency on healthy aging.

Centers for Medicare & Medicaid Services, www.cms.hhs.gov, the operations of the Medicare and Medicaid programs. Also, www.medicare.gov, the official Medicare site, which contains comparisons of Medicare and Medigap policies.

Consumer Protection Agency Senior Help. www.usa.gov/Topics/Seniors/ Consumer.shtml, Web page with links to consumer information specifically for senior citizens, including information about a wide range of topics, from buying cars to saving money.

Department of Health and Human Services, www.hhs.gov, includes links to many of the department's agencies.

Eldercare Locator, www.eldercare.gov, U.S. service to find programs and supportive services to help people care for an older member of their family in their homes and communities.

Medicaid, www.cms.hhs.gov/medicaid/consumer.asp, home page for Medicaid consumers.

Medicare, www.medicare.gov, home page for Medicare consumers.

Medicare Nursing Home Compare, www.medicare.gov/NHCompare/home .asp, provides detailed information about the performance of every Medicare- and Medicaid-certified nursing home in the country.

National Aging Information Center of AoA, www.aoa.gov/naic, this link skips the Administration on Aging introductions and such and goes right to the information for seniors.

National Institutes of Health, www.nih.gov, provides links to several institutes, including the National Cancer Institute and National Institute of Diabetes and Digestive and Kidney Diseases.

National Library of Medicine; Senior Health, www.nlm.nih.gov/medlineplus/ seniorshealthgeneral.html, gathers health news about seniors on a daily basis.

Social Security Administration, www.ssa.gov, everything about Social Security and its many services.

Local Resources

Religious
Consult a religious organization, such as:
Catholic Charities Family and Community Service
Jewish Community Services
Federation of Protestant Welfare Agencies
Arab American Institute
Buddhist Association of the United States

Organizations
Salvation Army
American Red Cross
Mental Health Association
Legal Aid
Council on Aging
Long-Term and Assisted-Living Facilities

Agencies and Government Organizations
Area Agency on Aging (AAA)
Commission on Aging
Department of Health
Department of Housing
Department of Human Resources
Department of Social Services
Department of Welfare
Eldercare Locator
Health and welfare agencies
National Long-Term Care Ombudsman (locate through your closest Area Agency
on Aging; aoa.gov)

BOOKS

Hayden, Joanne S. *Surviving the Home*, Joanne S. Hayden, 5202 S. St. Rd. 421,
Zionsville, IN 46007.

Kane, Robert, and Joan West. *It Shouldn't Be This Way: The Failure of Long-term Care.*
Nashville: Vanderbilt University Press, 2005.

Mace, Nancy L., and Peter V. Rabins. *The 36-Hour Day: A Family Guide to Caring
for People with Alzheimer's Disease, Other Dementias, and Memory Loss in Later Life.*
4th ed. Baltimore: Johns Hopkins University Press, 2006.

Marriott, Hugh. *The Selfish Pig's Guide to Caring: How to Cope with the Emotional and
Practical Aspects of Caring for Someone.* London: Polperro Heritage Press, 2003.

McCullough, Dennis M. *My Mother, Your Mother: Embracing "Slow Medicine," the Compassionate Approach to Caring for Your Aging Loved Ones.* New York: HarperCollins,
2007.

McLeod, Beth Witrogen. *Caregiving: A Spiritual Journey of Love, Loss, and Renewal.*
New York: John Wiley, 1999.

Sabel, Martin R. *The Elder Care Survival Guide.* Silver Sage Publishing, 2008.

Sankar, Andrea. *Dying at Home: A Family Guide for Caregiving.* Baltimore: Johns
Hopkins University Press, 1999.

Woodson, Cheryl E. *To Survive Caregiving.* West Conshohocken, PA: Infinity Publishing Co., 2007.

Acknowledgments

I have a great many people to thank for their help in creating this book. I especially want to recognize all the hard work that Jeannine Ouellette did in making the book more accessible to people. Dan Buettner has been a strong and constant supporter, giving me good advice about how to communicate better and ultimately helping me find an agent. That agent, Marly Rusoff, believed in this project and stuck with it. The editorial staff at Avery has been consistently upbeat and gave me lots of latitude, even when I insisted that caregiving was not always a happy topic. Ted Fishman gave me good advice about my writing.

My sister, Candy, and my wife, Rosalie, shared their caregiving insights with me. We lived through many caregiving experiences together. Rosalie read an earlier version of the manuscript and made a number of observations. Tom Laehner provided valuable drug information.

When I wanted to illustrate this book with real-life stories other than my own, I turned to Professionals with Personal Experience with Chronic Care (PPECC), a group I had started after writing a book about my mother. I put out a call to members of the group and the response was gratifying. Many had great stories to tell. I specifically want to thank Lyndon Drew, Riley McCarten, Kathleen Coen Buckwalter, Elanne Palcich, Gayle Kvenvold, Sandy Walls, Christine Costa, Carole Howey, Joann

Howitz, Eville Gorham, and Eric Haugen. Two people were especially generous with stories and insights from their own caregiving experiences. Deb Paone and Shirley Barnes spent time with me and commented on the manuscript, as well as providing many of the quotes used in the book. The Saint Therese Home graciously allowed me to reproduce several tables from their book, *The Complete Guide for Senior Care*.

Index

organization and record-keeping, 26, 101
seeking medical information, 101–2
by government or agency employee, 41,
207, 208–9, 249–50, 251
by professional
as client's employee, 250–52, 254
hospital discharge advocacy, 217–18
locating and hiring, 252–53, 313–14
objectivity and knowledge, 94, 217–18,
248–49, 253–54
selection of nursing home, 282–83
See also advocacy and involvement
cataracts, 136
catheterization, 150, 202–3
CCRCs (continuing care retirement
communities), 262, 263–64
certified home health agencies (CHHAs), 226
choking risk, 121, 203–4
Chronic Care (AARP), 87, 93–94
chronic conditions. *See* ailments and chronic
conditions
CLASS (Community Living Assistance
Services and Supports), 59
clutter, 124, 126–27
cognitive impairment. *See* Alzheimer's disease;
dementia
community-based services
caregiver support and assistance, 23, 243, 247
Medicaid coverage for, 55, 59
private long-term care insurance for, 59
Community Living Assistance Services and
Supports (CLASS), 59
compassion fatigue. *See* burnout and exhaustion
confusion
Confusion Assessment Method (CAM),
174–76
delirium, 173–76, 196
hospital-induced, 173, 196, 199, 200
medical conditions causing, 78, 152–54,
179, 182
medications causing, 155, 168
sundowning, 200
See also Alzheimer's disease; dementia
conservatorship, 32
constipation, 151, 154
continuing care retirement communities
(CCRCs), 262, 263–64
costs. *See* money matters

daily living. *See* ADLs (activities of daily living)
day care
adjustment to, 111, 246–47
adult day health centers, 246, 261, 264–65

for dementia patients, 110–11, 246–47
as long-term care option, 261
death. *See* end-of-life care
debilitation, 206, 219–21
dehydration, 153–54
delirium
causes, 173
versus dementia, 173–74
hospital-induced, 173, 196
recognizing, 173, 174–76
dementia
behavior management, 168–69, 189
behavioral changes, 185
causes, 186–87
clinical patterns, 187, 188
day care for, 246–47
versus delirium, 173–74
driving impairment, 116, 117–18
drugs exacerbating or mimicking, 163
drugs to treat, 168, 169, 188–89
genetic factors, 187
guardianship, 32
illnesses exacerbating, 185–86
incontinence, 151, 152
memory and executive function loss,
184–85
pain and, 185–86
preparation for, 187
risk tolerance, 29–30
seeking help, 238
sexual activity, 131
specialty clinics, 188, 189
stress of dementia caregiving, 189–90
summary of advice, 192
sundowning, 200
wandering, 30–31
See also Alzheimer's disease
depression
of caregiver, 105, 109, 114
of older person
loss of appetite, 123
medication for, 159
in nursing home, 293
recognizing, 156–58
self-neglect, 126
diarrhea, 152
diseases. *See* ailments and chronic conditions;
Alzheimer's disease; dementia
divestiture, 57–59
doctors
in case management, 26, 80, 82–83,
96–98, 100
changing, 84

advocacy for residents, 36–38, 277, 292
availability, 280–81
benefits to patient and caregiver, 40
care planning, 292–93
choosing, 279–81, 282–88
complaints against, 11, 34–35, 37–38
comprehensive geriatric assessment by, 86–87
convenience, 279
cost, 281–82
doctors at, 84–85, 277
as failed option, 293
family councils, 38
Green Houses, 276
history of, 274–75
hospital discharge to, 210, 212
hospitalization by, 196–98
as long-term care option, 260
Medicaid coverage, 55–56
Medicare coverage, 47, 224
moving to, 288–91
moving to different facility, 35, 280
Nursing Home Compare, 280, 282, 314
poor communication by, 277
quality assessment, 282–88
redesign and reform, 16, 275–76
rehabilitative care, 224, 225
for respite care, 247
sedation of patients, 168
sexual activity at, 131
summary of advice on, 294
visits to residents, 35, 292

osteoporosis, 139–40

PACE (Program of All-Inclusive Care for the Elderly), 264–65, 314
pain management
analgesics, 170–72
constipation caused by pain medication, 151
for dementia patient, 185–86
hospice and palliative care, 261, 298, 300
during rehabilitation, 222
Palcich, Elanne, 35
palliative care, 261, 262, 300–301
Paone, Deb, caregiver observations
caregiver's self-care, 105, 107, 113
checking on caregivers, 243
cooking and meal-planning by older person, 120
discussions with doctor, 122
getting help, 23, 107, 242
managing medications, 95
transportation of older person, 118

Patient Protection and Affordable Care Act
of 2010
income eligibility for Medicaid, 54
long-term care insurance, 59, 62
Medicaid funding for community-based care, 55, 59
payment for Medicare Advantage plans, 52
prescription drug coverage, 48, 48n8
spousal protection in Medicaid eligibility, 56
patients' rights, 208, 209, 313
physical restraints, 144
Physician Orders for Life-Sustaining Treatment (POLST), 71
physicians. See doctors
planning
advance directives, 68–75, 296–97
avoidance by older person, 27–28
care financing, 59–64, 65–67
estate planning, 57–59, 64–68, 253
hospital admittance, 198
long-term care decisions, 40–41, 210–17, 258–59, 272
for nursing home care, 292–93
risk tolerance, 215–18
political advocacy, 306–11
POLST (Physician Orders for Life-Sustaining Treatment), 71
prescription drugs. See medications
primary care doctors, 79–80, 84–85
privacy
bathing, 24, 124–25
health records, 100–101
toileting, 35
private long-term care insurance, 59–62
Program of All-Inclusive Care for the Elderly (PACE), 264–65, 314

QALYs (quality-adjusted life-years), 309

rehabilitation
advocacy and involvement in, 222
assessment of program, 221
assistive devices, 223
after hip fracture, 141
in home health care program, 225–26
Medicare coverage, 46–47, 213, 223–26
in nursing home, 224
options and combinations, 212–13
pain management, 221–22
in rehabilitation unit, 224–25, 260

rehabilitation *(cont.)*
    in skilled nursing facility, 225
    after stroke, 183
    types of therapies, 222–23
respite care, 110–11, 244, 245–48
retirement communities, continuing care
        (CCRCs), 262, 263–64. *See also*
        assisted-living facilities (ALFs)
reverse mortgages, 63–64

safety
    assistive devices and innovations, 223
    devices to summon help, 31
    "granny cams," 230–31
    of home environment, 30,
        126–30, 142
    Web resource, 313
Selfish Pig's Guide to Caring, The (Marriott), 109
sexual activity, 130–31
Shiffer, James Eli, 32
skilled nursing facilities (SNFs), 225
sleep problems, 155
Stevenson, David G., 1
Strauss, Peter, 16
stress
    of caregiving, 38–39, 104–6, 190, 235–37
    emotional strain, 17–18, 107, 109–11,
        189–90, 238

exhaustion and burnout, 38–39, 45, 105–6,
        110, 238
    guilt and anxiety, 107, 109, 232,
        238, 245
    of hospitalization, 7, 173, 193–94, 196
    older person's response to, 134, 153, 179,
        201, 204, 220
strokes, 180–83
supplemental insurance, 50–51
support for caregiver. *See* caregiver support
support groups, 111, 313

Taylor, Liz, 17
therapy. *See* rehabilitation
36-Hour Day, The (Mace and Rabins), 189
toileting, 35, 149, 150

urinary incontinence, 147–51

Vial of Life Project, 73–74, 312
viatical settlements, 62–63
vision loss
    diseases causing, 136–37
    home lighting and, 127
    safe driving ability, 116

wandering, 30–31
weight loss, 120, 123, 154